caring for

DONOR FAMILIES

before, during, and after

Also By Alan Wolfelt

Creating Meaningful Funeral Experiences:
A Guide for Caregivers

Creating Meaningful Funeral Ceremonies:
A Guide for Families

Death and Grief: A Guide for Clergy

Healing the Bereaved Child: Grief Gardening, Growth
Through Grief and Other Touchstones for Caregivers

Interpersonal Skills Training:
A Handbook for Funeral Home Staffs

The Journey Through Grief: Reflections on Healing

Understanding Your Grief: Ten Essential Touchstones
for Finding Hope and Healing Your Heart

Companion Press is dedicated to the education and support of both
the bereaved and bereavement caregivers. We believe that those
who companion the bereaved by walking with them as they journey in
grief have a wondrous opportunity: to help others embrace and grow
through grief—and to lead fuller, more deeply-lived lives themselves
because of this important ministry.

For a complete catalog and ordering information, write or call:

Companion Press
The Center for Life and Loss Transition
3735 Broken Bow Road
Fort Collins, Colorado 80526
(970) 226-6050

www.centerforloss.com

caring for

DONOR FAMILIES

before, during, and after

Raelynn Maloney, Ph.D.
Alan D. Wolfelt, Ph.D.

Companion
PRESS

An imprint of the Center for Loss and Life Transition

Fort Collins, Colorado

Companion Press is an imprint of the Center for Loss and Life Transition, 3735 Broken Bow Road, Fort Collins, Colorado 80526.

Printed in the United States of America.

17 16 15 14 13 12 11 10   5 4 3 2 1

ISBN: 978-1-617221-36-1

To the thousands of families who have enriched our lives—and the lives of so many others—by allowing us to companion them before, during, and after their donation experience. We are humbled by your strength, your generosity, and your compassion.

CONTENTS

Foreword 1
Introduction.. 5
Before: Caring for the Family from the Beginning 11
Co-Creating A Meaningful Experience 11
Understanding The Family's Initial Responses 12
The Special Immediate Needs of the Donor Family............. 18
   Physical Needs 19
     Nourishment/Bodily Care...................................... 19
     Nearness to the Person 20
     Physical Safety 20
   Emotional Needs... 21
     Time with the Injured Person................................. 21
     Time Alone... 22
     Permission for Emotional Expression 22
     To Observe "Good Care".. 23
     To Take an Active Role 23
     Guidance or Permission to Do the Unthinkable 24
   Cognitive Needs... 26
     Information About the Injury, Prognosis,
     and Declaration of Death...................................... 26
     Information in "Doses"... 26
     Choices and Options... 26
   Social Needs.. 27
     Supportive Presence... 27
     Support from Other Bereaved Families....................... 28
   Spiritual Needs... 29
     Make Use of Ritual... 29
     Embrace Faith... 29
     Question Beliefs... 29
Helping Families Understand Brain Death 31
   Talking With—Not At—The Family 31
   The Brain Death Conversation................................ 32
   Explaining Brain Death....................................... 33
   Enhancing the Family's understanding of Brain Death........ 37
     Barriers to Understanding Brain Death 39
     Barrier #1: Overcoming doubt and distrust.................. 39
     Barrier #2: The language barrier 42
     Barrier #3: The emotion barrier.............................. 43
     Barrier #4: The assumption barrier 45
Exploring Options and Choices 47
Continuing Your Care 50

During: Caring for the Family through the Donation Experience 55
Initiating the Donation Discussion: The Art and Science 56
From Functionary to Facilitator:
Beyond Consent to Genuine Support 57
Components of the Donation Discussion 60
   Timing of the Discussion 60
   Location of the Discussion 61
   People Involved in the Discussion 62
Structuring the Discussion 65
   Familiarizing yourself with the family 66
   Structuring the discussion 67
   Offering information 68
   Answering questions 69
   Summarizing 70
Decision-Making at the End-of-Life 71
   End-of-care decisions 71
   Considering autopsy 72
   Choosing a funeral home 73
   Deciding when to leave the hospital 73
Responding to the Family's Decision:
Honoring Family Choices 74
Leave-taking: Honoring Final Moments
with the Person Who Has Died 76

After: Caring for the Family After the Donation 91
Emphasizing the Donor Families:
The Importance of Honoring the Story 93
   Empathy Means Being Involved in the
   Feeling World of Donor Families 95
   Empathy Means Not Trying to "Fix Things"
   for Donor Families 96
Dispelling Misconceptions About Grief 96
   Misconception #1: Grief and mourning are the same 96
   Misconception #2: There are predictable, orderly
   stages to grief 97
   Misconception #3: We should avoid the painful parts
   of grieving 97
   Misconception #4: We should "get over" our grief as soon
   as possible 98
Unique influences on the grief Experience 98
   The Circumstances of the Death 98
      Sudden and unexpected death 99
      Premature and untimely death 99
      Stigmatized death 99
      Violent and traumatic death 101

The Nature of the Relationship with the Person who Died... 100
The Unique Characteristics of the Bereaved Person 100
The Unique Characteristics of the Person Who Died 101
The Family's Religious and Cultural Background 101
The Ritual or Funeral Experience 101
Common Responses to Grief and
"Companioning" Helping Roles..................................... 103
Shock, denial, numbness and disbelief 103
Disorganization, confusion, searching and yearning 103
Anxiety, panic, and fear.. 105
Physiological changes 106
Explosive emotions.. 107
Guilt and remorse 108
Loss, emptiness and sadness..................................... 109
The Six Reconciliation Needs of Mourning...................... 110
Need 1. Acknowledging the reality of death. 112
Need 2. Embracing the pain of loss............................. 112
Need 3. Remembering the person who died. 113
Need 4. Developing a new self-identity. 113
Need 5. Search for meaning. 114
Need 6. Receiving ongoing support from others. 115
Reconciling Grief 117
Development of a Family Support Project: A Working Model... 119
Phase One: Determining Needs.................................. 120
Phase Two: Establishing a Vision 122
Phase Three: Program Development............................ 125
Phase Four: Selecting Resources and Materials 128
Phase Five: Program Implementation and Evaluation 131
Self-Care for the Caregiver... 132
The Bereavement Caregiver's Self-Care Guidelines.......... 133
The Joy of Mini-Vacations 134
Work Smart, Not Hard... 135
Build Support Systems 138
Remember the Importance of "Spiritual Time"............. 139
Listen to Your Inner Voice 140
A Final Word... 143
A Bill of Rights for Donor Families 145
National Directory of Organ and Tissue Organizations 149
National Bereavement Organizations and Support Groups 151
Author Workshops and Trainings 153

FOREWORD

Eighteen years ago, I suffered the sudden death of my six-year-old daughter, Katie. Our family made the decision to donate her organs and tissues. For many years following her donation, we were left to grieve alone. We did not know any other donor families. We were sometimes ostracized by bereaved people who were not donor families, including, at times, our own family members and friends. Even some professionals distanced themselves.

In addition, follow-up information and communication was limited. Initial anonymous information about the organ recipients was provided, but updated information was almost nonexistent. Over time we learned that communication between donor families and recipients was frequently censored and sometimes not forwarded. Families who donated tissues were often treated as less important and had even more difficulty obtaining information and support. And when the programs were finally developed to assist families in the hospital, during and after the donation process, they were usually developed without input from those most intimately involved—donor families.

The National Donor Family Council, founded by donor families, grew out of these unmet needs. Because of their advocacy, support and communication improved. Organ and tissue procurement agencies began to develop new follow-up programs and enlist the support of families to educate professionals and the public about donation. Donor family programs began offering support groups, bereavement aftercare, donor recognitions, speakers bureaus, advisory board positions, and improved communication and information about recipients.

Although these efforts have been positive, still today many donor families do not feel supported. They feel invisible. The "experts"—the donor families themselves—are typically not involved in program design. They are talked about, not talked to. They are protected, not empowered.

Caring for Donor Families has the potential to dramatically change and improve this situation across North America. Each section leads caregivers through a step-by-step process designed to educate and support the family in the most effective way during the entire donation process, from the family's first interaction with a healthcare provider through the consent procedure and in the family's initial bereavement. Whether you are a brand new nurse or coordinator or a seasoned veteran who has worked with many donor families, standards of care will be validated, advanced, or refined.

A loved one only dies once, and caregivers need to make it the "best death" it can be for the patient, the family, and the professional. *Caring for Donor Families* emphasizes the death and its impact on the family, not the consent for organs and tissues. It is about caring with warmth, compassion, and presence. It is about providing frequent, honest, and consistent information. Its about empowering the family to be a decision-maker. It is about giving the family the gift of time to be with the person who as died, to say I love you, and to participate in the person's care. And finally, it is about providing support for all of the end-of-life decisions that must be made, including organ and tissue donation.

As a caregiver, if you make the decision to "companion" donor families, to make the death of a loved one "the best it can be," then you will be a participant in one of the most intimate life experiences for both donor families and yourself. You will become a very important part of the history of donor families, and they will always remember you and your compassionate care.

Caring for Donor Families: Before, During, and After is remarkable. It is one of the first publications written by professionals who truly understand the donor family experience. The authors, Raelynn Maloney and Alan Wolfelt, affirm that donor families are the "experts" and that caregivers must "seek to learn from them instead of focusing on being the expert who is there to teach them." Donor families have spent years researching, identifying needs, and writing and speaking about those needs and how to most effectively meet them. Finally someone has really listened. As the authors acknowledge, if you enter into a relationship with these families, "it is a privilege and an obligation to make their experience as meaningful and satisfying as possible."

Maggie Coolican, RN, MS, CDE
Founding Chair, National Donor Family Council

INTRODUCTION

For years, donor families have tried to help us understand the uniqueness of their experience. Through their stories, they've shared their struggles, their sorrows, their joys, their fears, their disappointments, and their gratitude. Their stories have taught us about the special needs of bereaved families as well as how you as a caregiver can best support them during this difficult life experience, which involves not only the death but the possibility of donation as well.

As we've listened, we've learned from them that there is an integral relationship between the death experience and the donation process from the family's point of view. We've learned it is not an event or a linear process to these families. Rather, the time you spend with the family is an *experience,* and they will remember it for the rest of their lives. We've learned that memories of the donation experience color the family's grief journey long after they leave the hospital. We've learned that supporting the family through the death and donation experience is just as important as providing good care to the organs and tissues that are part of that precious person this family is mourning.

As a caregiver to newly bereaved families, you have an opportunity to leave an imprint on a very sacred, personal experience. This is an opportunity to co-create comforting moments with the family during the last days and hours they are spending with someone they love. This is an opportunity to give the family an experience that they will speak well of as they share their story with others.

This resource was designed to help you help families as they encounter the death of someone loved and are given the opportunity to make a decision regarding organ or tissue donation. In the pages that follow you will not find a step-by-step instructional guide for bereavement care. This book is also not a template for holding the most effective conversation with a bereaved donor family with the hope of gaining consent. The kind of genuine caring that families need and deserve does not come when you have a script that guides you on what to say or do. The kind of caregiving that this book will help you provide involves joining the family in their loss and co-creating a meaningful experience around that loss. With this kind of caregiving you will experience moments of uncertainty as well as moments of helplessness, as you come to realize that you cannot take away the deep pain that comes when someone loved dies.

It is our hope that this book will inspire you to truly be present to every family you come into contact with, to be aware of and attend closely to families' needs, and to create a satisfying and meaningful *experience* with the family regardless of how limited your time is with them. The primary purpose of this resource is to add to your knowledge about grief and transform what you intellectually know about grief into caregiving skills that give you a sense of comfort and competence while you are in your role as caregiver. This is a book about authentic caregiving. As an authentic caregiver you will find yourself focusing on creating "safe places" (emotional, physical and spiritual places) for families to begin their work of mourning during the donation experience.

Recognizing that you may enter the family's donation experience at any number of different points, we've organized this book into three sections: **BEFORE**, which covers the time period the family is first contacted about the accident or injury through the time of the notification of the death; **DURING**, which covers the time period of the donation conversation and family decision through the time that the family leaves the hospital; and **AFTER**, which covers the time period following the hospital experience.

Throughout all three sections, we challenge you to think of yourself as an advocate for and companion to the bereaved family. We challenge you to create ways to make the donation experience more meaningful, memorable, and affirming for families. We offer suggestions and tools to help you provide a memorable experience. To enhance your learning in these areas, we encourage you to be an active reader and to practice and personalize the ideas presented here.

We are proud to be involved in helping donor families during such difficult times in their lives. As caregivers we are dedicated to trying to make a difference in this area because we are aware that each of us integrates loss into our lives when we have the support we need to heal. The journey through grief leads to transformation. The art of caregiving is to learn how to gently and lovingly companion our fellow human beings in the journey so that transformation begins.

As you enter your helping role with bereaved families, may you find renewed strength, inspiration, and hope in these pages.

BEFORE: THE FIGHT FOR LIFE

Looking back, we now realize with stark clarity that if someone is going to receive an organ transplant, someone healthy and strong needs to die a sudden death and become a donor. And every donor has a family. On February 5, 1996, our sixteen-year-old son, Scott, was involved in an accident. There was no way to be prepared for what we would experience and continue to experience as part of our journey.

The fact that Scott was airlifted, with life support, to the county trauma center and that the first report we were given was that the doctors saw "no life" in him, never diminished our hope that he would survive. Even after eight hours of surgery to close up the facial and cranial wound, with our son non-responsive and on life support, we were showing the doctors snapshots of our handsome son, so they would know how to make Scott look normal again.

After about thirty hours of waiting, hoping, praying, believing he would not die, we were confronted with the term "brain dead." Two neurologists came to tell us that the State of California requires two doctors to sign off on brain death. Both of them were prepared to make that determination based on the latest CAT scan results. There was no explanation of brain death. There was no communicated respect of the relationship that would be changed forever.

Anger rose up within us. Anger that these doctors could be so detached and speak without emotion about ending the life of our son. Anger, rooted in confusion and ignorance of medical technology. Our anger had demands. We wanted proof that he was "dead." After all, he did not look dead. His chest rose and fell with each breath. His heart was beating. His hands were soft and warm to hold. He looked asleep. We demanded a blood flow test to determine that blood was not reaching the brain.

It was not until that final blood flow test was completed and the results showed that blood was not flowing past the brain stem that we knew. We knew intellectually that a brain without blood is dead. We wish we had been invited to watch the blood flow test. It would have helped us recognize the reality of what was happening.

Editor's note: Tony and Bonnie Redfern of Kingsburg, California, were so kind to share this story of their son's death and organ donation with us, which we in turn share with you at the beginning of each of this book's three sections. The Redferns can be contacted through the website of their nonprofit New Path Center at www. newpathcenter.org, by email at tony@newpathcenter.org, or by mail at P.O. Box 874, Kingsburg, CA 93631-0874.

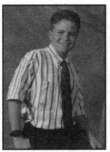

Scott William Redfern
November 23, 1979-February 6, 1996

BEFORE
CARING FOR THE FAMILY FROM THE BEGINNING . . .

As the family's journey begins, we, as caregivers, seldom realize the remarkable opportunity before us. Each time we enter into a helping relationship with a newly bereaved family, we accept their invitation to share in one of their most personal and deeply felt life experiences. Without even realizing it, we become a part of one of the most intimate experiences between the person who died and his or her family and friends. If we choose to enter fully into their experience, we have both a privilege and an obligation to make the moments they have with the person who has died as meaningful and satisfying as possible.

"Companion"

To companion someone who is bereaved means to walk with them, not in front of them or behind them. In fact, the word companion can be broken down into its original Latin roots: com for "with" and pan for "bread." Someone you would share a meal with. A friend. An equal.

Co-Creating A Meaningful Experience

Whatever your professional role (procurement coordinator, donor family coordinator, social worker, clergy, nurse, or physician), for purposes of this book and the subject matter covered herein, we are asking you to think of your role as one of *companion* and *advocate* to the newly bereaved family. In other words, it is your job to help them through the donation process and to make the experience as positive and meaningful as possible for them given these difficult circumstances.

If you are a companion to bereaved families, you seek to learn from them instead of focusing on being the expert. Yes, you may have the expertise to teach them about brain death, about their options for donation and about the recovery process, but it is they who will teach you what this death is like for them, what brain death and donation mean to them, what needs they have during their time at the hospital and beyond, and how you can truly help. This "teach me" attitude should guide every moment you spend with the family.

Companioning families can also mean helping transform the donation process into a memorable and meaningful experience. If you and your team work together to companion bereaved families, the family will feel respected and nurtured. They will discern that their thoughts and feelings truly matter, before, during, and after the decision regarding donation. They will not feel as if you were only interested in gaining their consent to donate. They may even invite a level of spirituality into this life-changing experience in a way they never have before, particularly if you help them make use of the leave-taking rituals discussed in this book.

Who Are Donor Families?

In the broadest sense, a "donor family" is any bereaved family who has made the decision to donate organs, tissues, or eyes from a family member who has died.

There are occasions when a family has agreed to donate but organs and tissues are not recovered or are unable to be transplanted. These families, because of their decision to donate, are also donor families. Despite the outcome of the donation, the families' intention and experiences that led them up to the donation decision is what creates a multitude of special needs that you as a caregiver can assist with.

Understanding The Family's Initial Responses

The family's journey begins long before they are recognized and referred to as a "potential donor family." The family begins their journey in a state of crisis, concerned and hopeful that someone they deeply love will pull through and survive no matter how horrendous the injury. From the moment they step into this experience with death, whether it is at the hospital or they are notified by telephone, each family deserves the supportive presence of caregivers who understand grief and the needs of newly bereaved families.

Those In Need

- *Currently, more than 108,800 people in the U.S. are waiting for a life-saving organ transplant.*

- *Every 10 minutes a new name is added to the national waiting list for organ transplants.*

- *An average of 18 people per day die in the U.S. while waiting for a transplant because an organ is not available in time.*

- *In 2009, an estimated 28,465 recipients received organ transplants.*

Those Who Give

- *Each year thousands of families are offered the option to donate the organs, tissues, and eyes of someone they love who has died.*

- *In 2009, approximately 8,021 families were able to donate their family member's organs for transplantation.*

- *These donations made by these families provided 28,465 patients with the organ transplants they needed.*

- *Some of these donor families are now survivors of suicide and homicide, which can complicate the families' grief process significantly.*

Sources: Coalition on Donation (www.shareyourlife.org) and United Network for Organ Sharing (www.unos.org), 2010

Regardless of how similar the circumstances, no two families will respond to crisis, trauma, and death in exactly the same way. Your ability to offer compassion and support to each family (and each family member) will depend a great deal on your personal awareness and beliefs about grief. Your beliefs about grief will influence the assumptions you make about the appropriateness of a family's reaction to various aspects of the death and donation process.

When you first encounter the family in the hospital, remember you are entering their lives at an incredibly difficult moment. Someone they love has just been involved in a sudden accident or has suffered an unexpected injury and is teetering on the brink of death. Does life get any harder than this?

Fortunately, nature has ways of helping people survive these exceedingly difficult moments. Shock and its cousins denial, numbness, and disbelief are nature's way of temporarily protecting people from painful realities. These normal, natural, and necessary feelings help people survive when life seems unbearable.

During this time you may hear families say things like, "I can't believe this is happening." "This can't be…I just talked to him this morning." or "This just seems like a bad dream." These types of statements are expressions of the family's shock and numbness. Through these responses, the family is teaching you that their emotions need time to *catch up* with what their mind has been told. During early discussions about their loved one's prognosis, for example, the family may initially push away the reality that the person may die. They may reside in complete and utter disbelief for hours.

Try These Supportive Helping Skills

- *Whenever possible, give the family members time to process this news and let the reality of the prognosis or the possibility of death sink in.*

- *Remember, numbness and shock are natural and help the family as they are trying to integrate the reality of this devastating loss.*

- *Don't try to hurry them in these early moments into leaving the hospital, making funeral arrangements, or making significant end-of-life decisions.*

- *We often want to help families through this by getting through it quickly, but what the family really needs is for you to simply be present and available to answer questions.*

- *Give the family permission to move along at a pace that will allow them to embrace this new reality, a reality that will change their lives forever.*

This shock and disbelief are often accompanied by feelings of confusion and an inability to concentrate. At times, you may find that you are answering the same questions again and again. The family may ask you to repeat basic information several times. They may forget your name even though you've told them more than once. Their attention may wander.

These are normal and necessary responses when the mind tries to process a new and devastating reality. It's as if the brain responds by becoming a filter, allowing drips of information in instead of a flood that might sweep away sanity.

Try These Supportive Helping Skills

- *Be patient with families who seem confused and unable to focus.*

- *Speak slowly and clearly, using simple language and short sentences.*

- *Repeat information as necessary without communicating the sense of impatience you may feel.*

The family's initial responses may also include anxiety, panic, and fear. Like most of us, they may fear death and its aftermath. They are often panicked about the prospect of life without the person they love. They may also be fearful of the machines that are keeping the body and organs viable as well as the experience of being within a hospital environment. Panic may set in when they realize that they may have to make the irreversible decision to remove the person they love from the "breathing machine" (the ventilator). For some family members, the body's autonomic nervous system also takes over, sometimes causing heart palpitations, queasiness, stomach pain, and dizziness.

Try These Supportive Helping Skills

- *You can help by being a calming and reassuring presence.*

- *Offer comfortable seating for the family.*

- *Bring them water.*

- *Take them outside for some fresh air if you think it would help.*

- *Let them know that these physical reactions are normal.*

Anger and other explosive emotions are common, too, among families in crisis. Because the injury may have been the result of a sudden and violent act, it is normal for some family members to be angry, sometimes extremely angry. Some of this anger may be directed at you or the hospital staff at times. Don't take this personally and help the family by being tolerant of their fluctuating emotions.

In an attempt to understand how and why this is happening, the family may feel the need to place blame. If the person was injured in a car accident, the family may have feelings of rage toward the drivers involved, for example. If the person attempted suicide, the family may be angry at the person or at themselves for having failed to prevent the act of taking one's own life (even though, as we know, they could not have). The family may also, at times, place blame on the healthcare team for not doing enough to save the person's life.

When a family expresses anger, you can help by listening without judging. This is difficult for many people because anger often makes us very uncomfortable. Feelings of hatred, resentment, blame, guilt, remorse, and regret are not bad or good—they just are. Allow the family to yell, sob, pace, or do whatever they need to do (without hurting someone else, of course) to release these powerful emotions. Explosive emotions must be expressed, not repressed. Don't ask the family to calm down or tell them that such expressions are inappropriate. Help them find the safest place to release these emotions openly.

Of course, profound sadness is at the bottom of all these emotions. While it can be difficult to accept the anger expressed by family members, it can also be difficult to bear witness to their pain in the form of sadness. Yet, as we will discuss in the AFTER section of this book, helping the family embrace the pain of the loss is a critical need of mourning. This is not a time to offer platitudes or use euphemisms in an attempt to blunt the pain.

DON'T SAY

- *He wouldn't have wanted you to be sad.*
- *You'll become stronger because of this.*
- *It was God's will.*
- *Crying won't make him come back.*
- *God only gives you what you can handle.*
- *Be glad you had him for so many years.*
- *He's in a better place.*
- *I understand how you feel.*
- *You can make meaning out of this through donation.*

DO SAY

- *I'm here to help in any way I can.*
- *Is there anyone I can call for you?*
- *Would you like to talk to a clergy person?*
- *The staff and I are here to help you.*
- *This is really difficult.*
- *I am truly sorry you are going through this.*
- *Is there anything you need?*
- *If I am giving you too much information at once, just tell me.*

You may feel profound sadness yourself as you spend time with bereaved families. As a caregiver you may vicariously experience some emotions that are similar to the families'. This is particularly true when the loss has some close associations to any of your own personal losses or life experiences. If you are feeling emotional, it's OK for you to express your sadness, to cry, to offer your sincere sympathy, to talk to coworkers and your family about your feelings.

To be empathetic to the grief of others means, on some level, to grieve the death yourself. Allow yourself to feel your feelings in the family's presence. They will sense your genuineness and trust will blossom. Be sure not so put so much emphasis on your feelings that it detracts from the family's experience. You may need to work through some of your own emotional experience with colleagues later, when the family is no longer present.

The Special Immediate Needs of the Donor Family: Physical, Emotional, Cognitive, Social, and Spiritual

The death of someone loved creates special needs for all families. Just as no two losses are experienced in exactly the same way, no two families will have exactly the same needs as they encounter the pain of losing someone they love. During this time, bereaved families not only grieve uniquely, they often *need* uniquely as well. The exclusive opportunity for some families to donate their loved one's organs, tissue, or eyes creates a new set of needs for the family during this death experience. As a caregiver, your sensitivity, knowledge, and skill in meeting these immediate needs is critical to the family's long-term response to grief.

While there may be some commonalities, each person will have needs that are as unique and individual as their grief. Naturally, there will be circumstances you cannot control that greatly impact grief responses, such as past loss experiences, past and present coping styles, availability of external support, and cultural/ethnic background (see the AFTER section for more on the uniqueness of the grief response). What you can control, however, is the sensitivity and compassion that is shown to families as they teach you what their unique needs are during this time. Your ability to recognize, normalize, and respond to a family's requests can greatly impact the overall donation experience.

You may find yourself with a family who has trouble articulating or is uncertain of their needs. Keep in mind that the impact of losing someone loved is felt on every level of their being—body, mind, and soul—and their needs during this time span each of these dimensions. Physically, they become weary; emotionally, they are overwhelmed; cognitively, they become confused; spiritually, they are questioning all they thought to be true.

Outlined below are several potential needs of families as they begin their grief journey. We remind you to look to the family to guide you toward what is most appropriate, comfortable, and essential to them during this time. As the family teaches you what is important to them and you help facilitate their requests, you begin to co-create what may become a very affirming and meaningful donation experience.

Physical Needs

Nourishment/Bodily Care—During this "before" time, the survivor is focused on the person who is injured or has died. Taking care of one's self naturally becomes less of a priority. As a caregiver, you have the opportunity to help by encouraging the family to listen to what their bodies are telling them—drink plenty of fluids, eat when they are hungry or begin to feel weak, rest when they tire. A change of clothes and a shower can make an incredible difference. If possible, make food and drink available in the waiting area or have a map available for them illustrating where they may find bathrooms, showers, vending machines, telephones, the cafeteria, outside sitting areas, play areas for children, local restaurants and hotels.

Proximity to the Person Who Died —The opportunity for closeness to the person who is injured or has died is important during this time. In your helping role, you may, when possible, make room for the family in a waiting area close to the medical care unit. Honor a family's need to see the injured person as soon as possible after they arrive. For many, this will allow them to let the person know or feel they are "there." Even after the initial contact, frequent visitation and permission to touch, hold, and talk to the person may help to meet this important family need.

Physical Safety—This need is particularly important for families who have been traumatized because they were involved in or observed the event that caused the injury or death. Meeting this need may mean providing protection from someone who has brought harm to the injured person, distance from the place where the event took place, or refuge from the media.

Take some time to reflect on additional physical needs a family may have and ways you might meet them.

Integrating Flexibility Into Your Care

In many ways, the expertise in helping lies within the bereaved individual, not in any prescribed checklist of needs. Such a list, as the one provided here, may be useful at times. However, it can also tempt us into prescribing the needs of families during the donation experience. The needs of families are dynamic and ever-changing. In your role as caregiver, we invite you to modify your care to accommodate the diverse nature of each family. Be flexible and willing to advocate for a family. The most important gift we can give a family as they begin their grief journey is the presence of a person who is willing to be their voice and mediate on their behalf in a setting that is foreign to them. Always stay conscious of the influences that can encumber you in meeting the unique needs of each survivor.

What are some of the physical needs I see that families have and what am I doing to help with these?

1. _____
   _____
   _____

2. _____
   _____
   _____

3. _____
   _____
   _____

4. _____
   _____
   _____

Emotional Needs

Time with the Person Who Died—It is a natural instinct for some families to need to be with the body. Spending time with the body can facilitate the integration of this new reality for the family. It can help make the unreal real. Some families may desire to stay at the bedside, while others may spend very little time in the hospital room. Respecting any decision made by a family and withholding judgment of those who choose to distance themselves from the person who died are ways of demonstrating compassion and care.

Permission for frequent visitation will create an open invitation to the family to spend the amount of time with the person that is right for them. Take time to discuss fears and concerns the family may have about seeing the person, particularly when you notice they are completely avoiding contact with the person who has died. Perhaps they are afraid of what they will see or that this will leave them with a disturbing memory. This may be an opportunity for you to offer some information and guidance. Providing a description of the hospital room, the condition of the body and the injuries, or accompanying the family into the room may be helpful.

Time Alone—Privacy is important during these intimate moments, and we must respect a family's need to be alone with the person as well as to be alone with themselves. Their ability to withdraw from the situation may lessen some of the distress they are feeling as a result of the multitude of sounds and activities surrounding them. Suggest a quiet, safe area where they can go for a while when they feel the need to escape.

Permission for Emotional Expression—The death of someone loved is an emotional experience, and families need a safe place to express emotions during this time. It would not be unusual to see family members crying, hugging, shouting, arguing, and even laughing at times. The family may spend time reflecting on the life of the person, his personality, his interests and his accomplishments. For some, emotional expression will be reserved for times when they are alone, while others will find comfort as they mourn in the presence of family, friends, and caregivers. Help the family to find a place that feels safe for them. Safe havens for the expression of emotion might include the chapel, a private waiting room, or the patient's bedside. When expression is not done here, but instead in a more public area such as the hallway or the nurses' station, we may immediately feel the need to quiet the person or family. Recognize that quieting a family may be done out of our own fears or feelings of helplessness. However, when these bursts of intense emotion are disturbing to other patients and families, it is difficult to allow a family to continue. Remember, if you move too quickly to silence the family, you may send the message that their behavior is abnormal and extinguish their willingness to express these difficult emotions. Instead, honor the family's willingness to express their grief and pain. Help them to find a place where they feel less "exposed" while also reassuring them that their feelings are a natural response to this experience.

Observing "Good Care"—In the eyes of the family, "care" given to the injured or person who died includes not only the medical treatment received, but also the gentleness, respect, and concern shown to the body as medical treatment is provided. Family members seek reassurance throughout their time in the hospital that everything possible is being done to save the person they love. For some families, the monitors and equipment that fill the room make a clear statement that all efforts are being made. Other family members will find comfort in words of reassurance from nursing or medical staff. The body of the person who is injured or has died is sacred. Conveying respect, dignity, and compassion to the body even after the death has occurred (be it brain death or cardiac death) is important to the bereaved family. The gentleness with which you move or turn the person's body and calling the person by name are practical ways of demonstrating "good care."

When the patient is brain dead, the machines may be continued for a period of time while the family is making several end-of-life decisions. At this time, family members may be curious about the purpose of the machines and what appears to be a continuation of care being given to the patient after the person has been pronounced dead. Invite these questions. Although these will be answered in due time, when end-of-life options are discussed, take time to comfort the family with the gift of knowing the answers now.

Opportunity to Take an Active Role—Throughout the hospital experience, families may desire to participate in the care given to their family member. Feeling that they somehow are able to contribute and participate in the care may be important to some families. You may find that as you show them that it is OK to touch the person's body, brush her hair, or move her to a position that appears more comfortable, the family will begin to assist you and perhaps find new ways of demonstrating their love and caring for the person. Encourage families to participate in ways that feel comfortable for them. For some this may be taking an active role to start a prayer chain or asking questions of the physician and nurses that others are afraid to ask. Others will find it comforting to read to the person, assist with bathing or turning the person, or arrange the flowers or cards in the room. We have found that many families take comfort in observing or participating in "tangible rituals" that can take place during this time. Creating handprints, clipping a lock of hair, and gathering significant linking objects and placing them in a memory box are just a few of the rituals you can offer to families, regardless of the age of the person who died.

For some donor families, the decision to donate gives the family more time with the person's body. Organ donor families are often given additional time with the body while the medical team is completing their medical evaluation of the organs and locating potential organ recipients prior to the recovery. Not all families will choose to stay at the hospital during this time, but those who do need your continued support. At a time when there is little they can say or do to change the circumstances, there is often a high need to be "doing something useful." You may help the family to meet this need to take an active role by suggesting what other families have done during this time.

Guidance or Permission to Do the Unthinkable—Some of the families you encounter will have no experience facing the death of someone close to them. Never having done this before, they may at times need guidance or reassurance that what they are doing is appropriate and normal. Give them permission to do and say those things that need to be done and said. These may be some of the most difficult moments for you as a caregiver to witness. You may feel uncomfortable or uncertain of whether the wishes of the family are "appropriate" at the time of death. It may seem odd that a family wants to take photographs of the person who has died, hold or read to their child, or crawl into bed with their spouse. There is nothing wrong with holding on to this memory, this moment. Encourage families to embrace these moments and take opportunities to create final memories that they will carry with them for a lifetime. The greater injustice would be for us as caregivers to discourage or prevent them from engaging in these meaningful and comforting moments.

What are some of the emotional needs I see that families have and what am I doing to help with these?

1. _____

_____

_____

_____

2. _____

_____

_____

_____

3. _____

_____

_____

_____

Cognitive Needs

Information About the Injury, Prognosis and Declaration of Death—A family can only deal with what they know, not with what they don't know. Naturally, a family will desire to know what has caused the injury, how the injury is being treated, who is in charge of the care, and what the chance is he or she will survive. They will want to share this news with other family members and friends who are concerned and awaiting a call. When possible, be available to the family as they relay this information to concerned others. Perhaps the family will call on you to assist them with this task to ensure that what is being said is accurate and consistent. Your patience and openness during this time will also help the family as they slowly begin to acknowledge the reality of the irreparable injury, the unfortunate prognosis, and eventual death.

Information in "Doses"—Information is often a source of power for families during this time when they are feeling powerless and have little control over the care of the person, their emotions, and the outcome of the situation. You may be concerned that the family is receiving more than they can handle during a time of suffering and stress. Providing consistent and accurate information in "doses," clarifying information, and encouraging and answering their questions can all reduce the cognitive demands on families during this experience.

How will you know if a family is experiencing "information overload?" The family's capacity to take in information will depend on several factors: how quickly the process is moving, the number of staff involved in the patient's and family's care, and the on-site support system available to the family. Agitation, irritability, and frustration during conversations may signal that the family feels bombarded with information and is in need of a few moments (or hours) of respite.

Choices and Options—Many families may feel immobilized as they observe others caring for the injured or person who died. In an effort to reestablish some sense of control over the situation, ensure that each family is informed of all the options available to them throughout their time at the hospital. This includes options to help nursing staff, even in small ways, as they care for the patient. At the end-of-life this includes the family's option to donate organs, tissue, or eyes when appropriate, to withdraw ventilator support, to remain at the hospital until the recovery is completed, or participate in a meaningful leave-taking ritual.

What are some of the cognitive needs I see that families have and what am I doing to help with these?

1. _____

_____

_____

2. _____

_____

_____

3. _____

_____

_____

Social Needs

Supportive Presence— Families share and outwardly express painful feelings associated with the loss as they begin the work of mourning. Recognize that even as a family shares this intimate experience with you, you are not the "lone caregiver." Others around you also have the capacity to offer comfort, care, and support to the bereaved. As you allow and even encourage a family to invite others—extended family, close friends, clergy, and hospital staff—into the experience, you communicate that this is an acceptable and healthy way to cope with the painful loss. Grief and loss are not to be handled alone and in isolation. With your help, families can begin to experience the caring of others and the supportive love they have to offer during difficult moments very early in their grieving.

Support from Other Bereaved Families—When possible, a family may find comfort in connecting with another bereaved family during or after their experience with donation. A family who has experienced the heartache of loss and grappled with the decision to donate may be a source of comfort and hope. A newly bereaved family may find greater comfort in sharing fears, questions, concerns, and hopes with a family who has been where they are.

What are some of the social needs I see that families have and what am I doing to help with these?

1. _____

_____

_____

2. _____

_____

_____

3. _____

_____

_____

Spiritual Needs

Making Use of Ritual—Words cannot adequately express all that is felt as a family confronts and acknowledges the death of someone loved. Providing opportunities for families to participate in end-of-life rituals during this time will facilitate their need to outwardly express their grief. Ask them if they would like a chaplain or clergy member to be with them or to assist them in creating a leave-taking ceremony. Invite the family to integrate rituals that are culturally, religiously, and spiritually meaningful to them. Honor the bereaved family's need to create final, sacred moments with the person who has died. These moments may be spent as family and friends gather around the bedside to pray together. A family may desire time alone in which to invite one another to reflect and reminisce about the person who has died. A family may choose to engage in a silent ritual such as a candlelight vigil or a final precious hour holding the person in sacred silence.

Opportunities to Embrace Faith—Families enter this experience with a variety of beliefs about religion and spirituality. These beliefs often influence the family's view of death and donation. Allow the family to teach you what they believe about the afterlife or a higher power. Discover the ways in which faith beliefs influence their views of death and donation. If faith is important to the family, allow them to express it in ways that are appropriate and meaningful for them. Their beliefs may be much different than your own. Listen without judging. Remember also that having faith does not mean this family shouldn't hurt. Faith doesn't eliminate the feelings that accompany loss. Compassion and caring means providing opportunities for families to express their faith as well as their grief.

Permission to Question Beliefs—When someone loved becomes ill, is seriously injured, or dies, it is natural for families to question their beliefs about their safety in the world, life's purpose, the benevolence of a higher being, and the afterlife. Family members may displace feelings of anger on family, hospital staff, or God.

Encourage the person to talk about these feelings of anger, fear, and uncertainty.

There are so many questions and so few answers for the family. Often "why" questions will precede "how" questions posed by the family. The family may ask, "Why is this happening to us?" and "How am I ever going to get through this?" Faith-based questions such as "Is this God's will?" or "Is she with God now?" are not uncommon. There are no simple, straightforward answers to any of these questions. As caregivers, the most you can offer is a listening ear, an open heart, and a willingness to explore the questions with them

What are some of the spiritual needs I see that families have and what am I doing to help with these?

1. _____

_____

_____

_____

2. _____

_____

_____

_____

3. _____

_____

_____

_____

Helping Families Understand Brain Death

Understanding and acknowledging brain death may be one of the most difficult tasks for families during this time "before" organ donation is discussed. Although it is relevant only for families of potential organ donors, it is such an integral part of the donation experience that we feel it requires a great deal of understanding. As caregivers, one of the greatest challenges is helping families understand the finality of this type of death. In part, this is difficult because the family continues to see what appear to be signs of life even after they are told their loved one is dead.

Even the use of the term "brain death" may create confusion for families. Consider for a moment the young woman who is told her husband died suddenly from a heart attack (not from brain death). Everything was done in an attempt to save his life. She asks to see him, to say goodbye, and as she stands near his bedside, there is no mistake that this is his lifeless body and that he is no longer alive. By contrast, when someone is brain dead and on a ventilator, the heart continues to beat, the chest rises and falls, and the skin is warm to the touch. All the vital signs of life are present for hours, sometimes days following declaration of brain death. Is it any surprise that some families hold onto hope that the person will survive even after the diagnosis of brain death is made?

Communication skills during this time are critical as you try to help the family understand that when the brain dies, the person dies. The content of the conversation as well as the way information is presented can certainly impact a family's understanding. The brain death conversation is more than simply defining brain death for a family.

Talking With—Not At—The Family

Take a moment to reflect on a time when you witnessed a family being notified about the death of someone loved. Who did most of the talking? Did the family actively participate in the conversation? Often a great deal of miscommunication occurs when a family is talked at or talked to. Talking WITH rather than AT the family opens up a new door to communication. This allows you to facilitate ("to facilitate" literally means to "make easier") the conversation rather than dominate it.

As you begin to spend this time talking with survivors and allowing them to participate in the conversation, you will find that you learn more about a family's willingness to listen, their ability to comprehend what you are saying, and gaps that exist in their understanding. For example you might say to the family,

"I understand this is a difficult time for you. Because I haven't been here with you through all of this, can you help me understand what's happened with Paul since you've been here?"

Talking with the Family About Brain Death

You, like many caregivers, may be wondering where to begin with this conversation. Begin by reminding yourself that, unless you have spent every moment with the family, you can never be certain what information they've already received. Ideally, the team of caregivers (clergy, nurses, physicians, social workers, and procurement coordinators) has provided consistent and accurate messages to the family throughout their care. However, it is not necessarily what is conveyed to the family that is important; what is important is what the family has understood. Although we hesitate to offer you a detailed script (because each interaction with the family should be genuine and personal), we do provide you with several example dialogues to help illustrate the words that you might use.

If you truly are joining the family in their experience, you'll take time to discover not only what they've been told, but also how they understand what they've been told. For example, you might begin by asking,

"Can you tell me what you've been told and understand about Paul's injury?" or "Some of the physicians and nurses may have used the term brain death with you. Can you tell me what this means to you?"

For some families, it may be helpful to explain why it is important that they understand the concept of brain death. You might say,

"Brain death can be confusing for some families. It seems that during a time when nothing makes sense, it might be helpful if I can eliminate as much confusion as possible."

How families come to understand brain death and what is essential to their understanding of this type of death is not entirely clear. This makes it difficult to know what should be included in this particular conversation. We do know that using the same description of brain death with every family in no way guarantees that each family interprets the information in exactly the same way. The family's interpretation will be influenced by several factors, including their previous personal experiences, interactions with other staff, ability to comprehend, and willingness to accept what is being shared.

Remember, the family is experiencing shock, numbness, confusion, and disbelief during this difficult situation. As a caregiver to an emotional and distraught family, you also may be emotional during this time. Your comfort with this conversation may take some practice. With practice and experience you will likely find that it is necessary to adjust your style and the content of the conversation with each unique family.

Explaining Brain Death

In explaining brain death, caregivers must convey to surviving families two primary concepts. First, brain death is not the same as coma. Second, the heart and lung function should not be confused as life signs.

Brain death can be described as cessation of function of the entire brain, including the brain stem. While the higher centers of the brain are involved in cognitive function, the brain stem is involved in control of such bodily functions as temperature, cough and gag reflex, and breathing.

As you talk to the family, it is important to provide a simple, clear and concrete explanation of the make-up of the brain (higher centers of the brain and brain stem) and the function of each part. You may explain by saying,

"The cerebral cortex is the part of the brain that controls who we are and what we do. This outer part of the brain is what makes us walk, talk, and interact as a human. This area also controls consciousness. The inner part of the brain, the brain stem, is the part that controls those functions we don't have to think about on a minute-to-minute basis, such as breathing, pupil response to changes in light in the room, gagging or coughing when you get something in your throat and so on. This area controls these basic human reflexes."

A family may be more familiar with the term "coma " than brain death. There is a common misconception that coma and brain death are one and the same. As you know, they are not. Misunderstanding of these terms can often generate false ideas about the survivability of the person's condition.

Patients in coma have full or partial function of their brain stem. Simply stated, coma is loss of function of cerebral or higher centers of the brain. This loss of function may or may not be permanent. Other terms such as persistent vegetative state are often used interchangeably with the term coma. From the family's perspective, coma often implies that the patient will one day regain consciousness. In fact, some patients in a comatose state do regain consciousness, even after several years. This is possible because in coma, the brain stem continues to function at some level.

Being aware of this potential for misunderstanding, you may routinely say to families,

"Some families have asked me how brain death is different from a coma. They have heard stories about people in a coma waking up after six weeks, six months, or maybe even six years and they wonder, if they waited long enough, would the person somehow wake up. But Paul is not in a coma. There is a very distinct difference between brain death and coma. Coma means that only the outer part of the brain has been damaged. Remember, this is the area managing consciousness, walking, talking, and those kinds of behaviors. This outer area of the brain is made up of similar types of cells, and sometimes for people in a coma, the undamaged cells that remain can learn the function of the damaged cells and eventually take over. However, the cells in the inner part of the brain are so specialized that no other part of the brain can learn to do their job. Remember, this is the part that controls reflexes like gagging and coughing. So, when those basic human reflexes have irreversibly disappeared, we know they will never return. Some of the testing the doctors have been performing on Paul is designed to determine the presence of these basic responses to find out if the inner part of the brain has any function."

You might go on to explain that in brain death, there is massive swelling in and around the brain. This swelling is the result of the primary brain insult and is a normal body response to injury. Ultimately, if the brain swelling cannot be controlled, it increases to a point that it prevents blood from reaching the brain cells. Without blood flow, the brain cells are deprived of oxygen and cease to function. When this involves all cells of the brain, including the brain stem, there is irreversible cessation of brain function, or brain death. The loss of the brain stem function is what makes brain death different than coma. The entire brain is irreversibly destroyed. No one regains consciousness once brain death occurs.

As you explain the irreversible nature of the injury, it is important to convey to the family that the entire brain has stopped functioning because of the injury. This could be conveyed by saying,

"When people use the term brain death, they really do mean that the brain has died. The activity that once kept the brain alive is no longer there and there is nothing that the doctors can do to restore it."

The fact that the heart continues to beat after a patient is declared brain dead can cause a family great confusion. In explaining this concept, keep in mind the relationship between the brain, the heart, and the lungs. Envision these three organs as a circuit, with each one required to function in order for the other two to also function. If any one of these three ceases to function and is not replaced by a transplant or artificial device, death occurs. The circuit starts with the brain, which sends a signal to the lungs to take a breath. The lungs take in oxygen, which is sent to the heart for circulation to the rest of the body. The heart beats at the speed of its own pacemaker, with the only connection to the brain a nerve that instructs it to slow down. The heart takes the oxygenated blood and sends it to the brain. The brain cells use the oxygen to function, and send a signal to the lungs to take in more oxygen. And so the cycle continues.

It is well known that the heart can stop and death not occur. Every day hundreds of people have cardiac surgery where the heart is stopped and a bypass machine replaces it temporarily. There are people who survive with artificial hearts. If the lungs stop, a ventilator can take over the function of providing oxygen to the body. Theoretically, the ventilator can replace the lungs indefinitely. Unfortunately, when the brain ceases to function, there is no replacement.

It is important for families to understand that the ventilator is maintaining the lung function, and that the heart will continue to beat for 24-48 hours, as long as it gets oxygen. Surviving families should understand that the heart and lung function are artificial, and without the brain to guide all of the other bodily functions, even the machines will not keep the heart beating for long.

Families can understand brain death. It must be explained carefully and at the level they can comprehend. It is futile to describe brain death to the family using complicated medical terminology. Caregivers should be careful to avoid terms such as "life support" equipment, which may send a mixed message. Communication must include concepts that a family can relate to.

The explanation of brain death to a grieving family requires patience, good communication skills, reinforcement, and a thorough understanding of the subject matter by the caregiver. As the surviving family makes their grief journey, it would indeed be unfortunate for them to needlessly struggle to understand the death of their loved one due to poor explanation at the time of death.

Enhancing the Family's Understanding of Brain Death

Brain death is an abstract concept, and you may find it helpful to use some tools to add to the verbal descriptions and explanation being given to the family. Pictures or visual aids can often provide clarity that words alone cannot. At a time when concentration is compromised, visual aids provide a family with something to focus on, to refer back to as more questions arise, to react to, or to hold on to. Additionally, during this time a family may find it difficult to attend to only words. Pictures, drawings, or diagrams provide tangible, visual information about the brain's anatomy and the injury. Visual aids are available through the National Donor Family Council and UNOS.

Visual aids or images also serve a purpose for you as a caregiver. They can guide your brain death discussion and help you actively connect with the family. This conveys to a family that their understanding is important to you. As you interact, this "active dialogue" conveys to them that their ability to understand is important to you. The following sample dialogue is one example of how this can be done.

Using your hands, make a fist with your left hand and lay your right hand over the top of the left. I use my right hand to represent the outer part of the brain and describe the anatomy and function by stating,

"This is the part of the brain that controls who we are and what we do (referring to the right hand). This outer part of the brain is what makes us walk, talk, drink coffee, and interact as a human. This area also controls consciousness. The inner part of the brain, or my left fist, is the part that controls those functions we don't have to think about. It governs actions such as breathing, pupil response to changes in light in the room, gagging or coughing when you get something in your throat and so on. This area controls these basic human reflexes."

Occasionally a family may need more than drawings or diagrams to make the concept of brain death more understandable. If possible, consider offering the option of being present when brain death testing is performed. People can better understand what they witness or are a part of than what they've been told. It is often very helpful to let the family see some of the actual examinations to determine brain death. This might even include a family observation of the patient off the ventilator for a short period of time so they can see for themselves that there is no effort to breathe. This type of reinforcement of prior explanations can help the family greatly in their understanding.

Conveying accurate information concerning the time of death is essential. It can be confusing, even distressing, to families when the time of death on the person's death certificate does not correspond with the time of death given to them at the hospital. Be sure the family is informed that the legal time of death is at the completion of the second brain death exam.

The use of analogies and metaphors may also offer a more meaningful and sometimes more gentle image of brain death. One analogy that works well is the child in a swing. The caregiver describes a child in a swing, kicking her legs to make the swing go higher and higher. The child is the life in the swing. The child may jump out of the swing, leaving the swing without life in it. As we watch the swing, it continues its motion back and forth, but it continually slows and finally comes to a stop. The patient's body is analogous to the swing and once the life leaves it in brain death, despite all medical therapy, it will slowly and surely come to a stop.

Our sincere appreciation to Allan Davis, BS, RN, CPTC, Senior Organ Procurement Coordinator, MidAmerican Transplant, and Jodi Orlando, BS, RN, CPTC, Donation Specialist, Iowa Donor Network, for their contributions in developing this comprehensive and instructive review of talking with the family about brain death. As their words teach us, they have discovered the beauty of companioning donor families with compassion and patience during this most difficult conversation.

While analogies and metaphors have the capacity to produce clarity, they also can be misused and misunderstood by families. Be sure to test out any newly developed analogies or metaphors on your colleagues and friends before using them with a bereaved family.

Barriers to Understanding Brain Death

Doubt, distrust, language difficulties, emotions, and assumptions can create distance and interference as we talk with families about brain death. Here we'll explore each of the barriers in some detail and offer suggestions for overcoming these common communication barriers:

Barrier #1: Overcoming doubt and distrust by establishing trust and rapport

Every interaction is an opportunity to begin to build a relationship with a family. Whether you join a family the moment they step

Rapport Building Inventory

In an effort to assist you in exploring your facility's ability to foster trust and rapport with families, we invite you to make use of the following inventory. While this is not a scientific inventory, our hope is that you find it helpful in determining areas of strengths and weaknesses.

Responses are scored from 0 to 4: 0 = never; 1 = rarely, 2 = sometimes, 3 = most of the time, 4 = all of the time. Circle the number that most applies after each question.

Are families given consistent
messages by staff members about
the person's condition and about
brain death?   0 1 2 3 4

Is information on the person's condition
provided over time (in "doses") rather
than during a single conversation?   0 1 2 3 4

Are caregivers willing to adopt a "teach me"
attitude as they enter into the
helping relationship?   0 1 2 3 4

Are family members kept informed of
what the next step in the
care of their loved one may be?   0 1 2 3 4

Are caregivers open and honest about
what they suspect the outcome will be?   0 1 2 3 4

Are caregivers sensitive to and
accepting of the diversity among
families (i.e., religion, ethnicity,
socioeconomic status, etc.)?   0 1 2 3 4

Do caregivers share all they know with
families rather than
withholding information?   0 1 2 3 4

Are families' concerns recognized
and responded to immediately?   0 1 2 3 4

Are caregivers cautious about providing
any sense of false hope to a family?   0 1 2 3 4

Does the physical space surrounding
the family convey elements of
warmth and caring?   0 1 2 3 4

Do caregivers have the desire and
ability to connect with the bereaved
family (i.e., capacity for active empathy)?   0 1 2 3 4

Are caregivers patient with
families and mindful of the verbal
and non-verbal cues families
use to communicate?   0 1 2 3 4

Total Score: _____

*A score of 0 to 16 indicates that families are given little opportunity
to find trust and care in the presence of your staff and within your
facility's environment. We strongly encourage you to explore ways
your staff and facility can enhance communication skills and physical
surrounding. If you scored between 17 to 32, this is a good indicator
that families are surrounded by professionals who understand the
importance of establishing trust. However, your staff would benefit
from some additional training in the areas where scores were low.
Those scoring 33 or higher demonstrate very favorable perceptions
of their facility's interactions with families. Clearly, this is the type
of environment where a family is made to feel safe, cared for, and
understood.*

into the hospital or days into their experience, there is always opportunity to establish a connection with them. For some this ability to connect and build rapport comes quite naturally, while others must work harder in their interactions with the family.

Naturally, families will harbor some initial feelings of doubt and distrust as they find themselves surrounded by so much that is unknown and unfamiliar. Also, because brain death can be visually deceiving, caregivers must find ways to establish trust and rapport long before you sit down to talk about the death. Creating an environment where a family feels safe, cared for, and understood is essential to your role as caregiver. You can foster an atmosphere such as this by creating a physical space/environment that feels safe and comfortable, demonstrating directly that you care about how the family feels. You can also foster trust by offering open, honest, and clear communication throughout the process and being open to their inquiries no matter how intrusive these might be while you are doing others things.

Barrier #2: Overcoming the language barrier by using simple language

Language can create a number of problems when we examine it in the context of the brain death conversation. It is nearly impossible to control what information is exchanged and how it is conveyed as families communicate with a multitude of caregivers. You may not be the first person to mention the words 'brain death' to the family. In fact, the family may have contact with many nurses, physicians, clergy, and/or social workers long before your first encounter with them. Because of this, we strongly encourage you to discover what the family has already been told and, more important, their level of understanding of brain death. You might ask, for example,

"I realize it may be difficult to concentrate right now, so if something I say doesn't make sense to you, please tell me" or "As

I talk about this, what questions come to mind?" Your dialogue may include questions that allow you to check the family's perceptions, such as "Does that make sense? Am I making sense? Are there questions I'm not answering for you? Is there anything else you'd like to know?"

Obviously, newly bereaved families are under a great deal of stress. Their energy level will naturally be low, ability to concentrate impaired, and capacity to hear and understand compromised. Use language that a family can understand. Medical jargon can and should be translated into simple, clear, and concise language for a family. When possible, avoid using acronyms in your conversations with the family.

No matter how many families you've talked with about brain death, there is always room to enhance your skills. Each family you have the privilege of supporting is unique in more ways that we can begin to describe. While the general helping guidelines are intended to help prepare yourself for this conversation, we encourage you to be flexible in your approach with each family.

Barrier #3: Overcoming the emotion barrier by cultivating a willingness to participate fully in this emotional encounter

Providing a family with news of the death will likely be an intense and emotional conversation for both you and the family. Emotions and reactions during this conversation can dramatically differ

DO

DO organize your thoughts and ideas ahead of time. Practice your explanation of brain death. Explain it to colleagues, friends, or your own family as a means of making sure it makes sense to someone who may not understand. This will not only help you to organize your thoughts, but will also serve to build comfort and confidence when discussing the subject of death.

DO use the word death. This is essential in clarifying that brain death is death. Avoid commonly used euphemisms (e.g., passed away, gone, expired, etc.) in your conversation about the death. Work to become comfortable saying the words death and died.

DO embrace moments of silence. Know that it is okay to sit quietly with the family without exchanging words during this conversation. Try not to fill in gaps in conversation with meaningless words or explanations.

DO be patient. Allow the family to experience these moments and move at a pace that is appropriate for them. A family may prematurely verbalize understanding if they sense you are impatient with them.

DON'T

DON'T offer every family a "canned" explanation. Every family, every loss, and every grief experience is unique. The conversation will vary because each family brings with them their own set of previous experiences, values, and beliefs that impact which questions they ask and their ability to integrate some of the more technical information. In sum, work to adapt the content and style of your communication with each unique family.

DON'T do all the talking. As you "dose" the family with information, take care not to monopolize the conversation. Again, talk with, not at the family. Provide the family with plenty of opportunity to share in their own words what they've heard and how they understand this information. As you explain the circumstances, take a few moments once in a while to allow them to react to the information you've given.

DON'T rush through the explanation. Take time to truly be with the family. A family can sense when you are preoccupied and when you are fully present to them. If you have other things to tend to, be sure you not only allow adequate time to explain brain death, but also allow for questions and clarification.

among members of the family. Anticipate and respect a variety of emotional responses as you convey the news of the death.

Shock, confusion, panic, anger, sadness, and many other feelings are typical responses to the news that someone loved is dead. Collectively, we call these feelings *grief.* They are the feelings we experience on the inside when a loss occurs. To move on in their grief journey and to eventually reconcile this painful loss, bereaved families need not only to grieve, but also to mourn. Mourning is the outward expression of these grief feelings. In other words, it is letting grief move from the inside out.

In these early hours after brain death, it is your job to allow families to feel what they feel and to express those feelings—to mourn. When possible, give them some time to sort through their normal and natural emotions before moving on in the donation process. Be present to them and acknowledge the normalcy of their feelings. Bear witness to their pain without trying to take away their pain. Help them mourn and you will be helping them to reconcile the death of someone they dearly love.

As a caregiver, you may also experience feelings of apprehension and anxiety about conversing with a family who is visibly grieving. It is important that you provide a stabilizing, calming influence for a family during this difficult time. We encourage you to take time to center yourself before interactions with the family. A few moments of solitude or taking in several deep breaths may help to calm and relax you.

Barrier #4: Overcoming the assumption barrier by exploring general fears, concerns, and questions about brain death

An important and often missing piece to the brain death conversation is the active exploration of a family's fears and concerns. When you ask if they have any questions, they don't. Do not assume that by covering all of the essential information about brain death the family fully understands and acknowledges brain death. This

Involving Others in the Brain Death Conversation

Give survivors permission to invite others, including extended family, close friends, and children, into the brain death conversation. Perhaps some additional time can be spent helping those who will be offering longer-term support to the immediate family to understand the concept of brain death.

Cultural beliefs and values may also influence the next-of-kin's desire to invite others to be a part of this experience. As you become aware of family beliefs, traditions, or wishes, it may require extra effort on your part to accommodate requests that seem unusual. Perhaps this will mean finding a room large enough to accommodate the entire family during the brain death conversation or asking other professionals to assist you in talking with a larger number of family members about brain death.

will take time—much more time that you will have with them at the hospital. As a family begins to integrate this information, they will naturally be overwhelmed and need time and space for clarification and questioning.

You may find that some families have difficulty formulating questions or hesitate to ask certain questions, thinking them to be too basic or perhaps irrelevant. You have the opportunity to make certain that a family is not misinformed or feels their concerns are insignificant. Assure the family that as questions come up, you will be accessible to address them. Convey that no questions are off limits. Be prepared to jointly explore questions. Consider offering the family a resource that responds to commonly asked questions.

Where spiritual and faith-based questions are concerned, take care not to condescend or disrespect a person's spiritual values and beliefs. While you can't always offer concrete answers to difficult questions, you can listen and recognize and support feelings, concerns, and fears, no matter how unusual. If you feel they want more than you can give, you may wish to direct the family to a more knowledgeable resource, such as their religious leader, spiritual advisor, or hospital clergy.

Exploring Options and Choices

Earlier we explored the importance of moving the family toward an understanding of brain death. Naturally, once you feel you have provided all the information, answered questions, and addressed concerns, you are ready to move forward once again. However, simply giving all the information about brain death does not ensure that the family is ready to move forward.

Frequently, following the brain death conversation (and at times during the brain death conversation), newly bereaved families are immediately offered the option of donation. Unknowingly, caregivers bypass a very important phase in the donation experience. They do not take time to carefully explore with the family all of the options and choices available.

Have you ever felt the need to move yourself and the bereaved family quickly forward? This is a painful time, and it is never easy to witness pain and suffering in another. You may want the family to get through this painful experience as quickly as possible. Perhaps you feel that offering donation is the only good that can be found in this experience because other families may have taught you that they felt comforted knowing they could help others through donation.

If you quickly move through the conversation concerning end-of-life options, you deprive the family of the opportunity to slow down and begin to integrate this experience into their reality. Resist the temptation

The Concept of 'Uncoupling'

It has been suggested that by uncoupling (also referred to as decoupling or separating) the brain death and donation conversations, families have the time they need to begin to integrate the concept of brain death. However, some families may not allow you to separate the conversations, inquiring immediately following the death about the possibility of donation. Remember to be flexible in your interactions with the family and follow their lead. Allow them to teach you why it is important to them to move quickly into the donation conversation rather than diving into this simply because they brought it up.

to move the family quickly away from the pain they naturally feel after the brain death conversation by hastily offering options and choices. Find comfort in sitting with them in their pain. Wait. Be patient. Don't rush.

Often we mistakenly believe that the family who is ready to move forward quickly is "handling things very well"—much better than the family who requires more time and more patience. Respect survivors' needs to stay still or even turn back for more questions, fears, and concerns to be addressed before moving forward. Some will need more time to take in what's been shared, will want more time with the person who has died, or will need permission to escape from the unit for a while. Follow their lead and allow them to teach you what they are ready to understand and accept.

On the other hand, because we cannot predict the sequence or flow of the information families receive from other care providers, there may be instances when options are mentioned to a family before the brain death conversation. And occasionally a family will initiate a conversation about donation before you have talked to them about brain death. When this occurs, your instinct may be to pull the family back to the appropriate "phase" or "step" in the protocol. We urge you to resist this temptation to redirect the family. It is impossible to take back information that has been shared with the family. This may only create confusion and frustration. Telling a family "You're not ready to hear this yet" or "It's not the right time" may leave them feeling anxious, irritable, or puzzled. They may simply desire to know if this is a decision they should be prepared to make.

By disregarding their need for information, you risk jeopardizing their trust in you. Instead, be flexible and go where the family leads you. Resist the urge to master the situation and allow them to be your guide. This means you may need to talk with the family about brain death even before the person meets brain death criteria or is pronounced dead. In this situation the doctor and healthcare team should openly share what they anticipate will happen over the next several hours (i.e., the person will progress toward brain death).

Collaboration between the hospital staff and procurement agency seems necessary so that the most accurate information regarding donation may be conveyed to the family. In some cases, the person may not meet the medical criteria for donation, eliminating this option for the family. When a family initiates the discussion early on, the reasons can be conveyed to the family at this time.

The Family's Readiness

How can you be certain the family is ready for this next phase in the donation process? You may have learned that the most appropriate time to offer end-of-life options to potential donor families is after they understand and have begun the process of accepting the reality that brain death is death. But brain death is not a simple notion to grasp, especially during an emotional and fatiguing experience.

Because a family's understanding of brain death is often not the same as the caregiver's understanding, you may experience some ambivalence about proceeding. For example, a family may rely only on the physician's word that the person has died and show very little interest in a detailed explanation about testing, or how the brain works. Another family may express their understanding that the person is so severely incapacitated that they would "never want to live this way."

In both of these situations, the family believes that the person they knew and loved is no longer there, no longer alive. This is the real indicator of the family's readiness to start really considering donation (even if they have already brought it up earlier). Although a family's understanding is imprecise, they may accept that the person they knew is no longer alive and be ready to move forward. Uncertainty and ambivalence about the death as final are often present with newly bereaved families. Their grasp on the reality of the death will be apparent in the words and behaviors they display as they interact with you, with other family members and with the person who died. Watch, listen, and let them teach you where they are with this.

Continuing Your Care

Bereaved people have six important needs they must meet if they are to go on to reconcile their loss and to live and love fully again. The needs are discussed in the AFTER section of this book, for they are primarily tasks undertaken after the decision to donate has been made. But the first need of mourning—acknowledging the reality of the death—gets underway the moment the family receives the dreaded news that someone they love is near death.

Once brain death has been thoroughly explained to them and all their current questions have been answered, the donor family may begin to truly acknowledge the reality of the death. We say truly because, up until this point, denial is often stronger than the powers of reason. As we have pointed out, even after the declaration of brain death, the family may continue to deny the reality and to hold out hope against hope that the injured person will "wake up" and return to normal. Or they may vacillate between accepting and denying the reality.

Meeting this first need of mourning is a Herculean task. Try not to get angry or impatient with families who seem unable to move beyond this step. Consider how you might feel if your child or sibling or best friend was the person lying there, still breathing, still warm to the touch, still appearing alive. Don't pressure or shame families who simply can't acknowledge the reality of the death in a timely enough fashion; they are doing the best they can.

Finally, keep in mind that donor families will first acknowledge the reality of the death cognitively, with their heads. The brain

Caring for Donor Families

scans and other medical tests, together with the medical staff's grim conclusions, persuade them that the person they loved is, in fact, dead. However, full acknowledgment of the reality of the death takes much longer. Only in the coming months and years will the donor family come to acknowledge the reality with their hearts.

Questions to ask yourself as caregiver:

Explore and describe the thoughts and feelings you experience when you are in the presence of a bereaved family.

What assumptions do you hold about families who are grieving?

What types of death have been experienced by the families you've supported (e.g., sudden, untimely, violent, etc.)?

Can you describe the stigma often associated with deaths by suicide and homicide?

How have you been able to assess other stresses that may be impacting the family during this experience?

How have families directly and indirectly communicated their needs to you?

Which emotions have you witnessed families openly express?

What are the support resources available to the family during this time?

How have the cultural beliefs and traditions of the family influenced their experience with the death and donation?

Reflect on a time when a family has tried to teach you about the person who died. What did they want to share with you? How did you respond to their need to tell their story?

What, if any, reservations do you have about allowing the family to be the "expert" in their experience?

NOTES

_____

_____

_____

_____

_____

_____

_____

_____

Take time to briefly summarize below the essential teaching principles you have learned from reading the BEFORE section.

_____

_____

_____

_____

_____

_____

_____

_____

DURING: THE NEED TO HAVE A POSITIVE EXPERIENCE

As we waited for the final blood flow test to be completed, we recognized that decisions would need to be made. No one from the hospital approached us regarding organ donation at this time. We asked our brother-in-law, who works in crisis intervention, to help direct our thoughts regarding potential organ donation. Realizing that the fight for life would not be won, our focus changed to a fight for value, that some good might come from our tragedy.

Once the reality of brain death was confirmed, we made our intentions regarding organ donation known to hospital personnel. Within an eerie few minutes, a representative from the donor network was introduced to us. It seemed he had been waiting in the wings. We were led into a makeshift conference room, cluttered with boxes, linens and supplies. You would think they would have had a special place to do this kind of sacred work. We asked our eighteen-year-old daughter, Amy, (who had flown in from college) and both our brother and brother-in-law to come in with us. The donor network representative asked the lead nurse to join us, too, as a witness.

Even though we believed this was what we wanted to do, when we were faced with the forms and releases, and listened to the discussion of how parts of our son's body would be given away, we became physically and emotionally anxious. As nausea flowed over us, the donor representative became aware of the physical changes taking place in us. He quietly and respectfully closed the folder and invited us to share our feelings, questions and concerns. Giving us the gift of time—to express our fears, to have our loss honored—gave us the security that this was our decision, and we were able to regain some control of our bodies and emotions.

Once the forms and releases were signed, our role in this decision was done. The hospital personnel did the rest of the work. We said our last good-byes to Scott. He was breathing. His heart was beating. He was warm to the touch. He even "reacted" to certain stimulus. Even so, we were told that his reactions were only spinal cord reactions and that they didn't mean anything. He was gone.

How we wanted to hold him one last time, but we were afraid we would somehow "hurt" the remaining life that was in him and somehow jeopardize the transplant successes. Instead, we said good-bye, kissed him and walked out of the hospital with the hospital staff looking on in quiet, somber respect. We drove home to an immediate empty-nest.

We now wish that we had been told of some possible options available to us during our leave-taking. We would have benefited by being told we could have spent some time with Scott's body after his organs were removed. We never knew about that option. We wished we had some final ceremony at the hospital to honor Scott's gift. We wish we could have met the doctors who performed the organ removals. We would have benefited from being more involved in the transplant process. We believe that having a different leave-taking experience may have helped us achieve reconciliation with the reality of brain death. We never saw our son "looking" dead. Unfortunately, we struggled for months with the issue of "Was he really dead?" We continued to struggle with whether or not we made the right decision to accept brain death.

DURING
CARING FOR THE FAMILY THROUGH THE DONATION EXPERIENCE

Once you feel the family has an appropriate understanding of brain death, it is time to move ahead, further into the donation experience. This is often a time of transition for you as well as for the family.

As a caregiver, you may naturally feel a sense of failure and disappointment in the inability of the medical team to save the person who died. How do you cope with these feelings? Perhaps, like many caregivers, you focus on the good that may come from this situation. Believing the family may find comfort by donating may make this transition a bit easier for you.

Donation can certainly bring an element of hope to us and to the family when all else seems incredibly hopeless. However, you may discover that as you become more attentive to the prospect of donation, the grief experience of the family becomes less central to care that is provided. Suddenly they are viewed as a "potential donor family" and their loss experience takes a backseat to the possibility of donation.

Throughout your time with the family, remember this: you are with them because someone they love has died. This death is the core of their experience throughout their hospital stay. The family began this journey as a family in crisis and the crisis does not end when the option of donation is presented. Especially for caregivers participating exclusively in this part of the family's experience, it is easy to forget that they are not only a "donor family," but they are first and foremost bereaved.

Initiating the Donation Discussion:
The Art and Science

While the donation conversation contributes to only a small part of the family's grief experience, the memories of that interaction can have a long-lasting impact. In addition, this interaction can have a dramatic effect on the family's long-term perception of donation and transplantation.

During this time, your role as caregiver is not simply to inform the family of options. Rather, it is to explore with them those options that feel right for them. This means advocating for the family, ensuring they are given every option, helping them make informed decisions, and fully supporting their choices. While you may not agree with their personal decisions, trust that whatever a family decides is what is best for them.

Caregivers and donor families come to this experience with a host of divergent beliefs. To provide sensitive and compassionate care to a family does not require that you believe what they believe. You need only possess the willingness to ensure that every appropriate option is offered, including donation, as well as the conviction that it is their freedom to decide and the capacity to support their choices fully. At times you may find it difficult to suppress your personal opinions about donation. When this occurs, do not hesitate to consider seeking help from other professionals in supporting a family through this experience.

Conversely, you may passionately support and endorse the good that comes from donation. Perhaps you have witnessed the comfort it has brought families or the joy it's given to a transplant recipient. Because of your enthusiasm, you may find that your exploration of end-of-life options focuses exclusively on the option of donation. While donation can provide a wonderful gift, we again remind you that every family has the freedom to choose what is best for them. For some, what's best is not to proceed with donation.

From functionary to facilitator: Beyond consent to genuine support

Often the donation process is illustrated as a fluent, structured, and sequential process in a diagram or flowchart such as the one below. Here, donation is depicted as a series of phases that move the staff and family closer to the desired outcome—family consent.

Step 1: Identification and Referral—at the time of death (prior to brain death, when a patient is neurologically devastated), all patients should be referred for initial evaluation by the procurement agency to determine whether organ, tissue, or eye donation is an option for the family.

Step 2: Approach/Consent—approach family with end-of-life options, including donation.

Step 3: Evaluation and Maintenance—medically evaluate organ stability and suitability; stabilize the patient's vital signs.

Step 4: Placement—allocate organs and mobilize recovery transplant team.

Step 5: Recovery—operating room recovery and preservation of organs.

Step 6: Follow-up—provide follow-up information to the healthcare staff and family regarding the donation.

Protocols such as this can potentially enhance family care by helping the caregiver gain comfort with the process. But often, as in the flowchart above, the needs of families are vaguely referred to, and the caregiver's tasks tend to focus on donation rather than family support.

Death, grief, and the donation process are anything but orderly and predictable. The needs of families are dynamic and ever-changing as you move through the donation experience. Because of this, we believe that the best care is offered when caregivers abide by the institution's protocol while also learning to facilitate the family's donation experience. When caregivers are able to go beyond acting as functionaries of the donation process to carrying out the role as facilitators, the family's experience can be dramatically enhanced.

To facilitate literally means to "assist or make easy." Just how do functionaries differ from facilitators in the donation process?

FUNCTIONARY

- *A functionary views the donation discussion as a set of tasks to be completed (e.g., describing what can be donated, and dispelling myths about donation, completing the consent paperwork, etc.).*

- *A functionary adheres to the donation protocol without considering the uniqueness of each family.*

- *A functionary views him or herself as the donation expert.*

- *A functionary extends their sympathy to newly bereaved families, but is unwilling to join the family in their experience.*

FACILITATOR

- *A facilitator values the donation discussion as an opportunity to be fully present to a family, discover more about the person who died, and connect with the newly bereaved family. A facilitator views every interaction as important and makes whatever time they have with the family count.*

- *A facilitator is adaptive to the changing needs, requests, and demands of the family. Facilitators make it a priority to join the family where they are and walk with them through this experience rather than take the lead.*

- *A facilitator has a beginner's mind. Facilitators have a willingness to be taught what this experience is like for this family, what they need, and what they perceive as supportive.*

- *A facilitator goes beyond sympathy and has the capacity and desire to feel active empathy. Facilitators allow themselves to enter into the families' feeling world without over-identifying with the family.*

Integration Practice

Take a moment to reflect on the various tasks, functions and roles you engage in during the donation process. We invite you to explore those that involve direct contact with the family and those that do not. As you review your list, ask yourself: How do these influence the family's experience? How can I transform these functions into opportunities to "facilitate" or make easier this difficult experience for bereaved families?

_____

_____

_____

_____

_____

_____

_____

_____

Now as you review your list, ask yourself: How do these influence the family's experience? How can I transform these functions into opportunities to "facilitate" or make easier this difficult experience for bereaved families?

_____

_____

_____

_____

_____

_____

_____

Components of the Donation Discussion

Every moment with the family is an opportunity to facilitate a meaningful experience—a chance to nurture the family, connect with them, and to create moments that will be meaningful to them long after they leave the hospital. It is not always easy to think about your time with a family in this way. The multitude of tasks in the donation process and mounting paperwork sometimes may move your focus away from the family. Pay attention and try to notice when this is happening for you.

When the consent becomes the primary focus, the support and care you provide to the family changes. For example, your perceived role with the family, your ability to identify the family's needs as a bereaved family, and the content of your conversations with the family will be guided by your primary objective: obtaining consent.

Let's explore how this may influence the donation discussion. A consent-centered donation discussion will differ in many ways from a family-care centered discussion. A family-centered approach is adaptive and flexible. Decisions about the discussion are made in the best interest of the family—not the staff, not the procurement agency, not the transplant surgeons, and not the recipients.

Below we outline key components in the donation discussion that, when integrated properly, have been shown to increase family consent—timing of the conversation, location of the discussion, and the professionals involved in the conversation. However, as you will see, when the best interests of the family are considered, these factors are also key ingredients to creating satisfying memories of this experience for the family.

Timing of the Discussion

When is the "right" time for initiating the donation discussion? The answer seems straightforward: after the family understands and accepts brain death. However, we remind you that understanding and acceptance can be difficult to assess. It may be unrealistic to expect a family to fully acknowledge and accept the reality of the death during your time with them. A caregiver taking a family-oriented approach would recognize that a family's readiness is contingent upon several considerations, including but not limited to the length of time they've spent waiting for information or answers, their confidence in the care that was provided, their understanding of brain death, and their access to sources of support. These considerations will help you to find the right moment to move forward with this family. With each family we encourage you to ask yourself: *For this family, when is the most appropriate time to begin the donation discussion?*

Location of the Discussion

Where is the "right" place to begin the donation discussion? Caregivers who desire to offer a family-centered approach will recognize that there is no single best place for this discussion to occur. As you consider where to have this conversation, recognize that the family is in an unfamiliar environment. They are in a state of shock and confusion. The family has likely been bombarded with information and in contact with a multitude of people.

Take some time to find a place that conveys feelings of warmth, comfort, support, and privacy. You may encounter a family who would like to hold this conversation at the person's bedside. This may be where they feel warmth and comfort, and it is important to honor this choice. If together you decide to have this discussion elsewhere, be sure to check out the room you will be using before leading the family there. Are there enough chairs and are they comfortable? Is there a table? (Sometimes the use of a table can make this conversation feel more like a business transaction than a personal interaction.) Is the room big enough? Is it too big? Is the door accessible? Is the room in a quiet area, away from the medical unit and crowded waiting rooms? Will you feel compelled to quiet the family if they become loud in this location? Can the door be closed for further privacy? Is there a means of indicating your desire not to be disturbed?

People Involved in the Discussion

Who should be involved in the donation discussion? First, let us consider who are the "right" professionals. If we consider the family's needs, this discussion should include professionals who are familiar with the family as well as the circumstances of the death, the donation process, facts about donation, the rights of patients and families, and the hospital donation policy. Seldom will one individual fit this description. When possible, this conversation should be a collaborative effort among hospital staff and procurement representatives.

Now let's turn to the family members who are present during this time. Who has the "right" to be present? Before you begin the donation discussion, take a moment to consider the influence of each family member's presence during the donation conversation then ask the legal next-of-kin whom they would like involved. Remember, this is a time when support is critical for the family. By eliminating certain individuals from the conversation because they are not the "decision-makers" or they may sway the family's decision, you are eliminating an important support resource for that family. Be sensitive to the family's need to involve whomever they turn to for support and guidance during difficult times.

Disunity among family members can create an additional obstacle to donation. Limiting the number of people present so the family won't be swayed by the objections of others is only one alternative. Another is to recognize that if a family chooses to have someone present, that person's opinion is obviously important to them now and likely will be important to them as they mourn their loss.

Caring for Donor Families

A Child's-Eye View of Donation

Imagine for a moment the donation experience through the eyes of a child. What does it look like? Witnessing the tears and pain of parents and other relatives. Feeling uncomfortable and unsure in the sterile, restrictive hospital environment. Finding it difficult to comprehend what the doctors or nurses are saying about the person they love. Knowing that it is not good news.

Children may be siblings, daughters, sons, cousins, or grandchildren of the person who has died. They too are a part of the newly bereaved family. They too will mourn the death of this person they dearly love. They will remember this hospital experience as part of their story. And they too are worthy of the same gentle, patient, and loving consideration that is offered to the adult decision-makers. Indeed, in some instances children will be invited by caring adults to play a central role in the donation decision.

Often we fear that talking about the death and donation may frighten or upset the child. During the donation experience your role may include calming these natural parental fears. You have the unique opportunity to co-create a meaningful and memorable experience for the entire family, including children. We hope you find the following suggestions helpful as you offer care to the child members of the donor family.

- Encourage parents to invite their children to be a part of the experience rather than "protect" them from it.

- Understand that the child's life will undoubtedly be influenced by this inconceivable loss.

- Allow the child to openly mourn this death with the family.

- Watch and listen to the ways the child is teaching you about her needs during this time.

- Give the child permission to see, touch, hold, and talk to the person who died.

- Allow the child to guide you in understanding what he would like to know during this time about the person's injury, the medical staff, death, donation, and the multitude of additional questions that may surface.

- Offer honest information and explanation in a manner that is developmentally appropriate for the child.

- When possible, create a space that is "child friendly," where the child can play with toys, read books, have the freedom to move about, or rest comfortably when she is sleepy. If there is a play area outside or a nearby park, encourage adults to escape for some "play time" with the child.

- Invite the child to participate in—perhaps even plan—leave-taking rituals.

Donation Discussion by Telephone

Perhaps you are being asked to approach a family over the telephone with the option of donation. While this is not the ideal circumstance for holding such an intimate, emotionally-charged conversation, it is the only option in some situations. Across the country, tissue and eye donation is offered as an option to families during a telephone conversation. Several of the guidelines outlined in the BEFORE section are applicable for caregivers offering "long-distance" telephone support to families (e.g., information provided should be accurate and consistent, it may be necessary to repeat information, do not try to move the family away from their pain). Here are a few additional guidelines that may also be helpful:

- *Converse as well as obtain consent. Go beyond asking the donation question to asking the family about their experience at the hospital, talk about the person who died, offer words of encouragement and support.*

- *Provide accurate and consistent information. You may find it necessary to repeat information so be sure the information given is consistent throughout the conversation.*

- *Check for the presence of social support. Verify there are supportive others available to be there with the family once your call is over and you are no longer on the line.*

- *Call back. Consider making more than one phone call to the family. After your initial call and donation conversation, call the family a few hours later to ensure all questions have been answered, to ask how they are feeling or check in with them about anything else they might need right now.*

- *Be supportive of choices made by each family. Families have a right to have personal thoughts, feelings and beliefs which will ultimately influence their choices about what they feel is best for the person who died.*

Assembling the Family for the Donation Discussion

Following are some guidelines that may assist you in helping the family decide who should be involved in this conversation.

Allow the family to decide. Privately ask the legal-next-of-kin whom they would like involved. The number of family present for the discussion will likely vary with the age of the person who died, type of death, the family's previous experience with death, and the family's cultural background. Remember, relatedness is not always a good indicator of the strength of the relationship between two individuals.

Children have a right to be present. Adults have a tendency to want to "protect" children from seeing or hearing anything that might disturb them. Many caregivers, as well as parents we've cared for, assume that children of any age should not be included in decision-making. However, we must recognize they are survivors too, and have a right to participate. Of course, this is not to say all children should be present. Careful consideration should be given to the child's age, their understanding of death, their relationship to the person who died, and the willingness of supportive adults around them to answer their questions openly and honestly.

Structuring the Conversation

How do you begin the conversation and what information does the family need to make this decision? You may find that starting the discussion can be difficult. After all, what do you say to a family who is grieving?

As you communicate with a bereaved family, what you say is not nearly as important as HOW you say it. What a family will remember about their donation experience is not the specific words exchanged but the compassion, concern, and care you convey as you interact with them. Through words, actions, and gestures, you can convey that your desire to be with this family is genuine.

Here we offer some general guidelines for structuring the content and flow of the donation conversation in a manner that conveys caring and genuine concern. Of course, these guidelines may be applied to any conversations you have with the family at any point in the donation process.

Get to know the family

Some caregivers have little contact with the family prior to the donation discussion. If this is your first interaction with them, take a few minutes before you meet the family to talk with the other staff who've been supporting them in this experience. Be sure to allow for time to introduce yourselves to one another during your initial encounter. Take time to talk with the family about the person who died and the care the person is receiving. You might ask how they are feeling or what their needs are before you begin.

What would you like the family to know about you? What information can you share that will help you connect with them both on a professional and a personal level?

_____

_____

_____

_____

_____

_____

_____

_____

_____

_____

Provide Anticipatory Guidance

Most families have never been in this situation before. You can ease the discomfort and uncertainty felt by both you and the family by providing a brief explanation of what will take place. This allows them to anticipate what is to come and what they can expect during the next 30 minutes to an hour (or whatever the length of time is that you are typically with a family). You might say,

"I would like to spend some time with you talking about your interest in donating Paul's organs and tissues. I realize you've been given a lot of information already and now I'm offering more. But it's important that all your questions are answered about this process before we go forward. I'd like to start by talking with you about some of the things you may have heard about donation and answer any questions you may have, then, if you're interested, I'll go over the forms necessary to make this donation happen, and help you understand what Paul can donate, how long everything will take, and what you could expect after the donation. If you have questions at any time, please don't hesitate to ask."

What wording have you used as a prelude to the donation conversation? How might you improve the way you typically handle this part of the conversation?

_____

_____

_____

_____

_____

_____

_____

Offer Adequate Information

How much information is needed and in what order should it be presented? During this time you may fear that the family is being bombarded with information. At the same time, you know that information can help restore a sense of control and comfort. What is most important is that the family is well informed about what can be donated, their freedom not to donate, and what will result following the donation. While you may find comfort in outlining what you will share with the family, recognize that meticulously following an outline can result in an approach that feels and sounds rehearsed.

Are there pieces of information that you or your staff may be overlooking but, if shared appropriately, would help families through the donation experience?

_____
_____
_____
_____
_____
_____
_____
_____
_____
_____
_____
_____
_____
_____

Answer All Questions

Are you presenting information or conversing with the family? One way to help create conversation will be to encourage families to ask questions as you convey this important information. Give them permission to interrupt you as you speak. Periodically, you might ask if they have any questions or if what you've said is clear.

Develop a list of common questions families have asked you during this time. Which do you have "good" answers to and which do you need to research or consider a bit more to feel comfortable answering?

_____

_____

_____

_____

_____

_____

_____

_____

_____

_____

_____

_____

_____

_____

_____

_____

_____

_____

_____

Summarize What Was Talked About

Whenever possible, offer a summary of what you've shared during this time. They may need time to take it all in, sit with it, discuss it, and question it before they can make a decision. Perhaps you can leave them a resource with information on common questions families ask about the donation process. At this time a family needs to know how much time they have to decide and where you will be available should other questions arise.

Practice summarizing the donation discussion. Write a paragraph or a list of key topics covered and points addressed. Write as if you were talking to the bereaved family.

_____

_____

_____

_____

_____

_____

_____

_____

_____

_____

_____

_____

_____

_____

_____

_____

_____

_____

Decision-Making at the End-of-Life

Now that you have an understanding of how to prepare for and begin this conversation, it is time to present the family with their options and support them as they begin to make several final decisions. You may wonder about the family's ability to make decisions during this time.

Without a doubt, the stress and trauma the family is experiencing will impact their decision-making. Their energy level will naturally be low, their ability to concentrate impaired, and their capacity to hear and understand may be compromised. You will find, however, that most of the families you encounter are by no means incapacitated and unable to make decisions for themselves and their loved one. You can assist them during this time by continuing to provide information, education, and support.

Outlined below are several of the decisions donor families are asked to make during this difficult time. While the first decision we review is primarily a choice for organ donor families, the others outlined are decisions families who choose organ, tissue, or eye donation will encounter as well.

Cultural Considerations

As you explore options and choices with a family, be aware of the influence culture may play on a family's decision-making behavior. A person's culture, ethnicity, and religion may influence their willingness to make a decision, their openness to certain choices, and their reliance on others for assurance regarding decisions made. Regardless of your knowledge about the decision-making process or beliefs of another culture, remind yourself that each person and each family is unique. Overgeneralizations about cultural groups can be dangerous and misleading. When in doubt, remember the "teach me" philosophy and allow the survivors to teach you how their culture enters into this experience.

End-of-care decisions

End-of-care options may include withdrawing the ventilator or continuing the ventilator for the purpose of donating the organs. Some institutions or healthcare teams may also offer families the option to continue ventilator support until cardiac death (even with ventilator support, the organs of a brain-dead person will slowly lose function). Remember, a family's choice to withdraw the ventilator or donate organs does not preclude the donation of other tissues such as bones, heart valves, skin, saphenous veins, tendons, ligaments, and eyes.

The following dialogue illustrates this piece of the conversation,

"I realize you have been given a lot of information since you've been here and now it's time to make some important decisions. If all of this feels overwhelming as we continue, just tell me and we can take a break.

There are several options for you to consider right now. One choice you have is to discontinue all medical support and let nature take its course. Remember, Paul's body can no longer breathe without the help of the ventilator because his brain is no longer functioning, so shortly after it is discontinued his heart will stop functioning.

A second choice to consider is donating his organs. Up to this point the doctors have been focusing on caring for Paul's head injury, so we would need to take a closer look at how the organs are working before we can be certain that Paul could donate. It's important to know that the ventilator would remain on during this time and continue providing oxygen and blood to the organs. It usually takes about 12 hours to do this evaluation and determine which organs may be able to be transplanted. During this time, I would be here with Paul and available to you if you choose to stay."

Decisions regarding an autopsy

While having an autopsy may be a choice for some families, in some cases involving litigation it may be mandated. For many survivors, offering an autopsy is essentially offering them an opportunity to find answers. While there is no guarantee that the autopsy will provide answers to all of the family's whys and hows, the findings may provide some evidence of the person's cause of the death or that a crime has been committed.

Decisions regarding a funeral home

The funeral home and its staff play a critical role in the planning and carrying out of a meaningful funeral. Their advice, their compassion, their attention to detail, and their willingness to help the donor family personalize the ceremony will greatly influence not only the funeral service, but, ultimately, the family's healing.

Make it your business to learn about funeral homes in your area. Visit the facilities and talk to the owners or managing funeral directors. Get a feeling for each funeral home's strengths and weaknesses. Talk to the hospital chaplain and other area clergy about their funeral home perceptions. Then, when it comes time to help families choose the funeral home that best meets their needs, you will be better prepared to offer a sound recommendation.

Decisions regarding when to leave the hospital

Donation can be a very lengthy process, emotionally and physically draining for families as well as caregivers. You may rationalize to yourself that the family needs rest, that they should focus on taking care of other arrangements, that there is nothing more here they can do, or that staying would only prolong their suffering. Listen to the family. Remember, the only people who know what is best for survivors are the survivors. Giving a family permission to stay or leave is the only way you will discover what is best for them. They will never be given this time again. For some families, the wait that occurs during the donation process offers a precious gift—the gift of more time with the person who has died.

Responding to the Family's Decision: Honoring Family Choices

Each family chooses what, at this moment in time, feels best for them. While you may not agree with each family's decision, it is important to honor their personal freedom to choose. Honoring family choices means offering information, education, and choices—and then respecting the family's decision.

For some families, this will mean choosing not to donate. Some families choose not to donate because they cannot bear the thought of the body being cut into. Some choose not to donate because they are simply unable to accept the reality of the death. Some choose not to donate because for them, medical intervention of any kind violates what they perceive as God's will. Some choose not to donate because they are uncertain of the person's own wishes regarding donation.

Sometimes caregivers are disappointed, even angry, when a family chooses not to donate. While these are normal and necessary feelings, expressing them to the family is inappropriate. If you truly think of yourself as a companion and advocate to the bereaved family instead of a consent-getter, you will accept their decision not to donate with empathy and equanimity. Companioning donor families is partly about bearing witness to their struggles; it is not about judging or directing those struggles.

For families who choose to donate, this is often a time when both family members and caregivers struggle with conflicting emotions, feeling both sorrow for the family's loss yet joy that this decision to donate may spare several other families the pain of loss. Naturally, the paradox of emotions that emerge during the donation experience creates special needs for both survivors and hospital staff. Often, the staff's own need for support and open communication about these feelings goes unrecognized.

Caregivers may wonder if it is disrespectful to the donor and their family to openly express positive emotions about transplantation and the potential recipients. This experience is filled with many bittersweet moments for both donor families and caregivers. Your fear of upsetting the family or showing disrespect for the person who has died may lead you to suppress natural feelings of excitement, curiosity, and hopefulness. How can you feel sadness about the death and, at the same time, joy for the families of the potential recipients?

Be aware that your emotions may be at odds with one another. You may feel uncertain about how you should react. This is a natural response, and we assure you that others are also experiencing this emotional confusion. It is important to respect the positive and negative expressions of the family as well as other caregivers. As you witness this struggle in yourself, the family, and other caregivers, take time to offer reassurance and validation that these feelings are normal.

Many families will choose to leave the hospital at this time. Some will choose to stay for a short time. Still others will remain until after the

Ten Freedoms for Bereaved Donor Families

- *You have the freedom to create a donation experience that is meaningful to you.*

- *You have the freedom to spend this time the way you feel is right for you.*

- *You have the freedom to ask friends and family to be present and available to support you during this time.*

- *You have the freedom to ask any and all questions of those caring for you and the person you love.*

- *You have the freedom to make decisions that are right for you and your family.*

- *You have the freedom to make use of ritual that is culturally and spiritually meaningful to you as you encounter this painful loss.*

- *You have the freedom to leave the hospital when you are ready.*

- *You have the freedom to embrace both the pain of your loss and the joy of giving another the opportunity to live.*

- *You have the freedom to receive compassionate, ongoing support following the death and donation experience.*

- *You have the freedom to affiliate and receive support from other donor families and transplant recipients in the months and years that follow.*

recovery of organs, tissues, or eyes. What can we do for a family who chooses to stay? Perhaps they feel a need to be sure things are being handled properly, to be sure their loved one is not alone, or they simply desire more time with the person.

Regardless of the family's donation decision, it is your role to continue to offer information, reassurance, and supportive presence until they choose to leave the hospital. Discover how they would like to spend this time. When someone we love dies, our final moments with the person are treasured for a lifetime. What are the memories they would like to make during these final moments and how can you help them make this possible?

Leave-taking: Honoring Final Moments with the Person Who Has Died

"When words are inadequate, have ritual."

–Anonymous

Most of life's most important moments are honored by ritual—baptism, birthdays, graduations, weddings, funerals. Rituals help us express our deepest, most profound thoughts and feelings when words alone fail us or seem inadequate. Rituals also lend structure and a sense of dignity, honor, and importance to special occasions.

At a time of death, ceremony helps family members and friends acknowledge the reality and finality of the death. Ceremony also gives donor families a forum for saying goodbye and a feeling of finality to the donation decision, giving them, in effect, a meaningful memory of the final moments in the presence of the person who is dying.

Without ceremony, on the other hand, there is no leave-taking protocol. When should the donor family leave the hospital? How do they say goodbye? How do they honor the transition from life to death? These are often awkward questions, spoken or unspoken, giving rise to painful and awkward moments and, later, painful memories.

As caregivers at this critical moment in people's lives, we have the opportunity to facilitate the leave-taking process. At your hospital, will it be an awkward, empty, even scarring process or will it be enriching, beautiful, memorable, and healing? The choice is yours.

In the BEFORE section of this book, we explained that the first need of mourning for donor families (and everyone in grief) is to acknowledge the reality of the death. On some level, this first need must be met quickly for families to give their consent to donate organs, tissues, and eyes. Only over time, however, will the family fully come to accept the reality of the death with their hearts.

The second need of mourning, discussed in more detail in the AFTER section of this book, is to embrace the pain of the loss. To heal, families must not deny or run away from their painful thoughts and feelings but rather move toward them and embrace them. As Helen Keller once said, "The only way to get to the other side is to go through."

Caregivers at a time of death can help families meet this need by being honest and direct; euphemisms such as "passed away" or "no longer with us" attempt to soften a blow that should not

Rituals at a time of death:

- *confirm the reality of the death.*
- *help us understand that death is final.*
- *allow us to say goodbye.*
- *encourage us to embrace our pain.*
- *help us remember the person who died and encourage us to share those memories with others.*
- *offer a time and place for us to talk about the life and death of the person who died.*
- *affirm the worth of our relationship with the person who died.*
- *provide a social support system for us and other mourners.*
- *help integrate mourners back into the community.*
- *allow us to search for meaning in life and death.*
- *establish ongoing helping relationships among mourners.*

Symbols to use in leave-taking rituals

Symbols are an important part of ritual, for they represent a myriad of thoughts, feelings, and beliefs. In leave-taking rituals, symbols such as the cross (for Christians; other faiths use other symbols), flowers, and candles—and, of course, the body of the person who is dying—provide points of focus for the family. Because they represent such profound beliefs, they also tend to encourage the expression of painful thoughts and feelings. Furthermore, symbols such as these provide the comfort of tradition. Their continuity and timelessness ground mourners at a time when all seems chaotic.

Symbolic acts, too, often enrich leave-taking rituals. When family members light a candle during the ceremony, for example, they are provided with a physical means of expressing their grief. When they hold hands and form a circle around the person who is dying, they symbolically emphasize their ongoing love and commitment even in the face of death.

Some common symbols include:

- *Candles—the flame can represent the spirit; also, for some, life's continuation after death*
- *Cross—faith, crossing from earthly life into the afterlife*
- *Cup—nourishment, abundance, faith*
- *Flowers—support, love, beauty, remembrance*
- *Water—source of life, cleansing, renewal, rebirth*

be softened. You can also help by enhancing your capacity to be present to people in emotional pain. When family members cry, scream, or beg, do you look away and leave the room or do you look them in the eye and offer your comforting presence? Leave-taking rituals also help families embrace the pain of the loss.

The third need of mourning is to transition the relationship with the dying person from one of presence to one of memory. Because the donation process literally involves the physical death of the family's loved one, we feel it is incumbent upon caregivers to acknowledge and honor this transition through ceremony.

Leave-taking rituals clearly demarcate the "Before" from the "After." Families understand that they are "with" the person who is dying for the last time and thus want these moments to be meaningful. They know that the next time they see the body it will no longer be breathing or warm to the touch but cold and lifeless. Without ritual, this awesome knowledge is almost too much to bear.

Caring for Donor Families

You and your staff may be unaccustomed to participating in (let alone leading) rituals at the hospital. A staff training may be in order to broach the idea and to integrate rituals into the organ donation process. Please do not forego leave-taking rituals simply because your hospital staff "wouldn't do it" or "has never done it before." Your hospital chaplain or area clergy are good resources for assisting in the establishment of leave-taking rituals. And listen to your heart—would families truly be helped by such rituals? Can you in good conscience send families away without at least offering to help coordinate a brief yet meaningful leave-taking ritual for them?

Also be aware of the spiritual and religious beliefs of each family before offering a particular ceremony or choosing a person to lead the ceremony. Families of faith are often best served by a clergyperson affiliated with their place of worship or denomination. Families without a specific belief system may be comforted by a secular ceremony such as the one included here or by simply joining hands, sharing memories and saying goodbye. Some families won't want to spend any time with the body or will reject offers to hold a brief leave-taking ritual. That's OK, too. Remember—your role is to advocate for and companion this particular family at this particular moment and to do what is right for them.

Ask your hospital chaplain to put together some thoughts or passages for use in leave-taking rituals. You might also assemble a ritual notebook, in which you and staff gather appropriate poems, ecumenical prayers, and other readings. This notebook can then be referred to by any staff member, family member, friend of the family, or clergy person asked to help facilitate or participate in the leave-taking ritual.

Music is also an effective and meaningful addition to leave-taking rituals. Consider assembling a set of CDs with appropriate instrumental or "spiritual" music. Or ask the family what music they find most comforting and healing. Favorite music of the person who has died is another good choice and may be easily procured with a quick trip to the local music store. Have available a portable CD player or iPod dock to play the chosen music softly in the background.

Sample Leave-taking Rituals

Following are two sample leave-taking rituals for use with donor families. The first is secular (although it does refer obliquely to life after death) and the second, actually a sample of readings, is definitely Christian. Keep in mind that these are but examples and that each family's religious and spiritual orientations should be carefully considered before you offer a particular ritual.

A Secular Ceremony

The "Circle of Love" ritual (adapted from Remembering Well: Rituals for Celebrating Life and Mourning Death *by Sarah York) usually takes place with the family gathered around the bedside of the dying person (or after the death). As those present gently place their hands on the person or on the bedside, a clergy member or other designated person begins the ritual.*

"(Name), we're here to hold you in a circle of love and light."

A pause is offered and family members are invited to share their feelings, memories, or express their love for the person who has died. Some will share things left unsaid to the person. Others will simply want to let the person know they are there and offer reassurances that they will be okay when this is over. Still others may use this time to express those things they will miss when the person is gone.

"Let's now share with (Name) a blessing, a prayer of release, a message of peace."

The following meditation can be read collectively by everyone present or parts can be assigned so that each person's voice can contribute to this loving rite of passage.

I am the wind, breathing in you and for you, blowing gently over you, caressing you.

I am the earth, holding you. Give me the weight of your body and relax into my arms.

Caring for Donor Families

I am the sun, warming you, melting away the cares of this world.

I am the mountain, always here for you, always here for you, always here for you.

I am a river, flowing through you— through your head, your neck, your shoulders, your arms, your body, your legs, your feet. I give you peace.

I am the ocean, rising and falling, giving you deep beauty and rest.

I am the sky, open space never ending, open space, vast and edgeless space, where you may float forever and ever.

I am the Light, the Light of eternal spirit. I am all around you.

I am in this world and in all worlds, for I am the Light of all being.

(all together): I am peace, I am spirit, I am love, I am life growing into new life.

Readings for a Christian Ritual

Following are passages, prayers, and rituals taken from various worship books and recommended by Chaplain Harold Sheer, Pastoral Services, University of Iowa Hospitals and Clinics, for use with donor families.

Before the organ/tissue recovery when the life-support system will be withdrawn:

> *God of compassion and love, you have breathed into us the breath of life and have given us the exercise of our minds and wills. In our frailty we surrender all life to you from whom it came, trusting in your gracious promises; through Jesus Christ our Lord. Amen.*

At the time of death.

> *Child of God, go forth in the name of God the Father almighty who created you: in the name of Jesus Christ, Son of the living God, who redeemed you; in the name of the Holy Spirit who was poured out upon you. May you rest in peace and dwell forever in the paradise of God. Amen.*

When a child dies:

> *Lord, God, as your Son, Jesus,*
>
> *Took children into his arms and blessed them,*

So we commit this child (Name) into your loving care.

Grant us the assurance that you have received this life,
which you gave,

and grant that when we stand before you

we might be as innocent and trusting as little children.
Amen.

A prayer for the child's parent(s):

Compassionate God,

Soothe the hearts of (Name(s)) and enlighten their faith

Give hope to their hearts and peace to their lives

Grant mercy to all members of this family

And comfort them with the hope

That one day we shall all live with you

Through Jesus Christ our Lord. Amen.

A Service of Blessing

(Adapted and in part reprinted from Occasional Services, copyright 1982, by permission)

Dear friends: It is our hope that you have received love from
other people during these days: may this love and the love of
God comfort you in the days ahead.

Like the Israelites, who struggled in their wilderness
wanderings, perhaps you too have struggled in various ways
in this large medical complex.

May God bless you in your wilderness wanderings and may
you do what you can to be a blessing to one another.

"The Grace of our Lord Jesus Christ, the love of God and
the Communion of the Holy Spirit be with you all." (11
Corinthians 13:14)

Romans 14: 7-9

None of us lives to ourselves,
and none of us dies to ourselves.
If we live, we live to the Lord,
and if we die, we die to the Lord;
So then, whether we live or whether we die,
we are the Lord's.

Caring for Donor Families

For this end Christ died and lived again,
that he might be Lord both of the dead and the living.

Prayers

Lord God, God of mercies and God of all Comfort: We thank
you for your care in this time of trial and sadness. Console
and comfort these your servants with the assurance of your
tender compassions and unfailing love; through Jesus Christ
our Lord.

O God, your beloved Son took children into his arms and
blessed them. Give us grace, we pray, that we may entrust
(Name) to your never-failing care and love, and bring us all
to your heavenly kingdom; through you Son, Jesus Christ our
Lord.

Merciful God, comfort your servants whose hearts grieve,
and grant that they may so love and serve you in this life
that, together with this your child, they may obtain the
fullness of your promises in the world to come; through Jesus
Christ our Lord.

We Will Remember Him/Her Ritual

Invite the family and friends present to form a circle. Gently
encourage people to sit quietly and reflect on the goodness of the
person who brings them here. Suggest that when they are ready
that anyone who wishes may share favorite memories of the person.
You can help them with this by suggesting they consider some of the
following:

How has (Name) touched your life?

Have there been special times you will always hold close to
you?

Do you have a favorite story about (Name) that you can share
with us?

The intention of this remembrance ceremony is to help begin the
long, painful process of shifting from relationships of presence to
relationships of memory. As the leader, you are simply yet profoundly
facilitating the very early beginnings of holding memories up and
taking grief from the inside to the outside. Your quiet, calming
presence will help anchor those present as they "story" the life of

this precious person. Keep in mind that those present feel lost in the dark. The process of translating their memories into stories helps them experience some glimmer of light and hope in the midst of their darkness.

Remember—encourage people to share memories, but never force them. Some people may share more than one story while others sit quietly and listen. Do not assume that those who stay quiet do not find value in this ceremony. Some people are in shock and unable to speak even if they want to. Obviously, use good judgment in when and if you would use this ceremony. If those present are in overwhelming pain or extreme shock, asking them to be expressive may overwhelm them and make them retreat from you. However, you will sense that some families want and need to "story." In our experience, even when one or two favorable memories are expressed, it helps all present begin to "dose" themselves with the painful yet necessary process of authentic mourning. You can conclude this time of embracing memories in a variety of meaningful ways unique to the needs of the family you are companioning. For example, you might use a meaning-filled song selected by the family, a prayer, a poem, a reading, or simply a moment of silence.

If you are an excellent listener, you can frame-up the memories expressed in a reflection of the qualities that those present have shared with the group. For example:

> As we conclude our time of remembrance, let us give thanks for (Name's) life.
>
> Thank you (Name) for being a wonderful _____ (e.g. mother).
>
> Thank you (Name) for your gift of compassion.
>
> Thank you (Name) for your gentle spirit.
>
> Thank you (Name) for your sense of humor.

Your intention is to summarize the good qualities expressed by the group and plant them in the hearts and souls of everyone present. Your sensitive companionship to this family will never be forgotten. You will help them make a new beginning as they remember the life that has been lived. As you support the family, remember the words of T.S. Eliot, who once said, "What we call the beginning is often the end. And to make an end is to make a beginning. The end is where we start from."

A Continuation of Life Ritual

A family may want to say a final prayer or share their thoughts regarding the gift that will be provided to transplant recipients through the donation. Through the Continuation of Life Ritual, you will co-create a sacred moment for families closely linked to the donation experience—a moment that will allow and encourage the expression of hope the family feels for the future recipients. The family may choose to share in this ritual during their final moments before the person is taken to the operating room or following the organ or tissue recovery.

Before gathering the family together, offer family members who wish to be a part of the ceremony a special invitation, time alone, and the tools (a small journal and pen that they can keep) to write their prayers, thoughts, and hopes for the recipients. At an appropriate time, ask family members to gather around the patient's bedside.

A clergy member or other designated person will begin the ritual by saying "We know that soon (Name) will touch the lives of several others through his/her gift and donation. As we turn our thoughts toward the recipients, let us take time to share our prayers, thoughts, and hopes for their future."

The journal can be passed so that each person is given the opportunity to share what they've written, or you may choose to select one person to read all entries in the journal as the others listen quietly. The ceremony may conclude with a special poem, a piece of music, or the following prayer.

(Name), today and with each day to come our heads and hearts will be filled with thoughts and memories of you.

Although you will no longer be physically present to us, a part of you will remain with us forever. You will continue to be with us through the stories we share and memories we hold close. Others will continue to experience you through your gift—a gift of life, of love, and of another tomorrow.

We will miss your loving touch, but you will continue to touch the lives of others in an extraordinary way by sharing a part of yourself with them. We will miss seeing your smile and hearing your laughter, yet we know that because of your gift other families will continue to share moments of laughter and joy.

May your presence continue to be with us for a lifetime as well as with each fortunate recipient...wherever they may be.

Once you begin offering and carrying out leave-taking rituals for donor families, you will find that certain readings, rituals, and music seem to work well for many. Certain clergy and staff members will have a natural gift for leading or participating in these rituals. And you will come to know, we are certain, that donor families will find much more meaning and healing in the donation experience.

Questions to ask yourself as caregiver:

For you, what do you use to measure your "success" during the donation process (e.g., consent, family satisfaction, staff responses)?

How do you "facilitate" the donation process for families?

In what ways have you witnessed the family's grief impacting their decision-making?

Describe ways that you have found to support a family after their donation decision. Does the type, amount, or style of your support change depending on the family's choice?

What events, people, or elements of the process tend to distract you from your role as caregiver to the bereaved family?

What leave-taking rituals have you observed when supporting families?

In what ways have you tried to co-create a meaningful experience for families during your time with them?

NOTES

Take time to summarize below the essential teaching principles you have learned from reading the DURING section.

_____

_____

_____

_____

_____

_____

_____

_____

_____

_____

_____

_____

_____

_____

_____

_____

_____

_____

_____

_____

_____

_____

_____

_____

_____

_____

_____

_____

_____

After: The Search for Meaning and Reconciling Loss

During the next few days we received calls from the organ donor network updating us on the progress of the organ transplants. Because of extraordinary circumstances, we also learned through the media of one of Scott's organ recipients. We started to hear a new vocabulary. There was talk of organ "harvesting" and that the "prayers of the recipient's family had been answered." Although the organ donor network personnel were kind and helpful, we found through the media that Scott had lost his identity. All of a sudden he was no longer human. He was now a "cadaver" with body parts available to needy people who had been waiting for an available organ. There was a spirit of celebration as each potential recipient moved up the list. What they didn't seem to recognize is that with each movement to be the next-in-line, someone died to make that happen. The reality is, when that donor died, the "cadaver" left behind a grieving and hurting donor family who lost a loving member of their family.

After the last transplant report came in, we waited for the responses of Scott's four recipients. Although we could not know the names and identities of the recipients, we were told that we could expect a note of thanks from them. We waited weeks, months, and years without hearing anything. We finally wrote a letter to the organ donor network asking if they had received any word from any of Scott's recipients. With our urging, the donor network encouraged one recipient to write a note of thanks. The network sent this one very special note of gratitude. It is the only one we received, and we cherish the letter even to this day.

All in all, our experience as a donor family was good, but it could have been more enriching for us, enhancing our memory of our last moments with our son. It would have been good to know the options that would have helped us on our grief and mourning journey.

AFTER
CARING FOR THE FAMILY AFTER THE DONATION

While we recognize that the decision to donate organs or tissues is a helpful way to give some meaning to a tragic death, we also believe that we have both an obligation and an opportunity to help family and friends of the donor in their grief experience. This section of the book is about a shared challenge, a shared human concern, and a shared hope—sensitively and compassionately supporting every family during this naturally difficult time.

Our experience suggests that few helping situations are more challenging—or more rewarding—than the opportunity to assist people impacted by tragic loss. At the end of a life, when words are inadequate, the heartfelt presence of a genuine caregiver is seldom forgotten.

You may have heard that "grief is a normal process," yet the reality is that most people who are experiencing grief benefit from information, education, and ongoing support. Our hope is that the information explored here will serve as a source of encouragement and practical help to those caregivers who seek an understandable framework in which to view their helping role with bereaved donor families.

The information contained in this section is not intended to make you an expert in the area of grief counseling. Often grieving families are looking for someone who will walk alongside them, not lead them; someone who will listen with their heart, not analyze with their head; someone who will "companion," not "treat" them.

While we do not yet, and we certainly never will, know all there is to know about grief and mourning, we do have a good start.

"Companioning" the bereaved

I have been a grief counselor and educator for almost three decades. While I received traditional training in psychology and earned my Ph.D., over the years I have come to understand that what grieving people need from caregivers like us is not to be "treated" (which is what I was taught in school), but rather to be "companioned."

I have taken liberties with the noun "companion" and made it into the verb "companioning" because it so well captures the type of counseling relationship I support. Actually, the word "companion," when broken down into its original Latin roots, means "com" for "with" and "pan" for "bread." Someone you would share a meal with. A friend. An equal.

Here are a few additional distinctions between treating and companioning:

> *Companioning is about honoring the spirit; it is not about focusing on the intellect.*

> *Companioning is about curiosity; it is not about expertise.*

> *Companioning is about learning from others; it is not about teaching them.*

> *Companioning is about walking alongside; it is not about leading or being led.*

> *Companioning is about being still; it is not about frantic movement forward.*

> *Companioning is about discovering the gifts of sacred silence; it is not about filling every painful moment with talk.*

> *Companioning is about listening with the heart; it is not about analyzing with the head.*

> *Companioning is about bearing witness to the struggles of others; it is not about judging or directing those struggles.*

> *Companioning is about being present to another person's pain; it is not about taking away or relieving the pain.*

> *Companioning is about respecting disorder and confusion; it is not about imposing order and logic.*

> *Companioning is about going to the wilderness of the soul with another human being; it is not about thinking you are responsible for finding the way out.*

— Alan Wolfelt

Clearly, no one resource will teach us everything there is to know about supporting donor families.

Your own personal perspective on death and grief will probably change and grow with each new loss you encounter (it certainly has for these two authors). Perhaps, through deepening your human capacity to make an empathetic connection with donor families, you can create a deeper sense of meaning and purpose in both your work life and personal life.

Remember—our shared hope is that this information will inspire you to reach out to donor families more readily, more comfortably, and more authentically.

Empathizing with Donor Families: The Importance of Honoring the Story

If your desire is to support donor families in their grief, you must create a "safe place" for people to embrace their feelings of profound loss. This safe place is a cleaned-out, compassionate heart. It is the open heart that allows you to be truly present to another human being's intimate pain.

Helping people integrate death losses means being present to them and observing them—companioning them. The notion of observance comes to us from ritual. It means not only "to watch out for" but "to keep and honor," "to bear witness." To care for and about donor families is to nurture souls as they do the hard work of mourning.

A central role of caregivers to bereaved donor families is related to the art of honoring stories. Honoring stories requires that we slow down, turn inward, and really listen as people acknowledge the reality of the loss, embrace pain, review memories, and search for meaning.

Honoring stories of pain and grief doesn't require you to be an expert. Actually, purporting to be an expert to a bereaved person is dangerous. Implicit in any model of who we think we are is a message to others about who they are. The more you as a caregiver perceive of yourself as an "expert," the more pressure there is on someone to be a "patient." The biggest impediment to providing support to donor families in grief is the distinction between "us" and "them."

A central arrogance in considering oneself an expert is the perception that one has a superior knowledge of someone else's destination in the grief journey. We can be present, watch, and learn, but we cannot direct or even guide.

So what can you do to support bereaved donor families? Hopefully, you can help them feel understood by a least one other person. As a compassionate caregiver, you can ask yourself, "How can I establish a relationship with the mourner that provides a safe environment wherein he or she feels free to express grief without fear of judgment, isolation, or abandonment?"

Below is an introduction to the art of communicating "active empathy" to bereaved donor families. The inherent attitude of active empathy is "Teach me about your grief and I will be with you. As you teach me I will follow the lead you provide and attempt to be a stabilizing presence." After all, the true healer and authority is within the person who is experiencing the pain of loss, not in the caregiver.

Unless you as a caregiver are able to adopt this "teach me" attitude, you are likely to make judgments about the mourner's experience. When a bereaved donor family member expresses some thought or feeling, a potential tendency is to make some kind of evaluative reaction such as, "That's right" or "That shouldn't be" or worse yet, "That's pathological."

Empathy vs. Sympathy and Identification

There are critical distinctions between sympathy, identification, and empathy.

All too often, people experiencing grief are related to with a sympathetic attitude. While there is nothing wrong with sympathy, mourners need more than this "I feel sorry for you" way of being. Sympathy can be defined as feeling a concern for someone else without necessarily being involved in a close, helping relationship.

Another helping attitude that is even more destructive than sympathy is identification. This attitude is conveyed by people who submerge themselves with a person in grief and try to take on their feelings for them. They might make comments like, "I know just how you feel." When over-identification occurs, the caregiver actually becomes destructive to the helping process. The last person bereaved donor families will do the work of mourning with are those who convey an attitude of over-identification.

If you can't avoid these kinds of judgments, you will probably not permit yourself to understand and be taught by the grieving donor family. In other words, you will be likely to "treat" them, not "companion" them.

Empathy Means Becoming Involved in the Feeling World of the Families

Empathy requires the ability to go beyond the surface and become involved in the donor family's feeling world. To have empathy for people in grief does not constitute the direct expression of one's own feelings, but rather focuses exclusively on the person you are helping. In other words, communicating empathy to the mourner means to strive to understand the meaning of his or her experience rather than imposing meaning on the experience from the outside.

"Active empathy" means you are trying to grasp what it is like inside for the grieving person. What is the inner flavor and what are the precisely unique meanings that the person's experience has for him or her? What is it that she is trying to express and can't quite say? Perhaps the most complex, vital, and fundamental quality for caregivers to donor families is the capacity to convey "active empathy."

Empathy Means Not Trying to "Fix Things" for the Families

The value of the companioning, "teach me" attitude is that it takes the pressure off you as a caregiver to "fix things!" After all, you cannot take the pain away. Grief is not a disease you are trying to cure. However, you can help donor families become active participants in their healing.

You can help them embrace the six needs of mourning, discussed later in this section. You can help them feel understood and supported. You can allow yourself to be taught and follow their lead, dictated by their needs, not yours. Our choices about attitudes related to how to help grieving donor families often seem to relate to motives and needs. Adopting empathetic attitudes of "teach me about your grief and I will be with you" means you will have to be humbled by the experience and give up the status and power of being the all-knowing "professional." However, doing so will probably allow you to discover the unfolding of your "natural compassion."

Dispelling Misconceptions About Grief

As you prepare yourself to support donor families in their grief, we believe you will find it helpful to review some common misconceptions about grief. Providing heart-centered care to these families requires an understanding of these misconceptions. Don't condemn yourself or others if, as you read this section, you realize you may have internalized some of the misconceptions. Instead, make use of any new insights to help you become a better "companion" to those families you are privileged to help.

Misconception #1: Grief and mourning are the same.

As we pointed out in the BEFORE section of this resource, grief and mourning are terms that do not mean precisely the same thing, although most people use them interchangeably. Actually, grief is the composite of thoughts and feelings you experience within yourself about a loss. Mourning, on the other hand, is the external expression of that grief. Crying, talking about the person who died, journaling, and celebrating special anniversary dates are just a few examples of mourning. To heal, donor families must not only grieve, they must mourn. You can help by providing ongoing forums in which it is safe for them to mourn.

Misconception #2: There are predictable, orderly stages to grief.

You probably learned about the "stages of grief" somewhere in your schooling. Popularized by Elisabeth Kubler-Ross in her landmark text *On Death and Dying*, the stages of dying were later extrapolated to cover the stages of grief: denial, anger, sadness, acceptance, yet they were never intended to be used to describe the grief experience of bereaved families. While grief often manifests itself in these ways, and at times there is a logical progression of emotion, grief is not predictable. It is tempestuous and fickle, revisiting its earlier emotions without warning, bounding here and there, sometimes skipping "stages" altogether. Let the bereaved donor family teach you about their grief without imposing any sort of structured order or attempting to move them "forward" in their grief journeys.

Misconception #3: We should avoid the painful parts of grieving.

Our society often encourages prematurely moving away from grief instead of toward it. The result is too many bereaved people either grieve in isolation or run away from their grief. Far too many people view grief as something to be overcome rather than experienced. When people avoid the pain of grief, they avoid healing. Instead, it is your role as caregiver to help bereaved donor families find ways to slowly embrace the full force of their pain so that someday they can again embrace happiness.

Misconception #4: We should "get over" our grief as soon as possible.

No one ever "gets over" the death of someone loved. Instead, we learn to make it a part of our lives. We learn to live with it. You cannot help bereaved donor families "get over" their grief, but you can help them work through it and learn to reconcile themselves to it. With reconciliation, which typically takes years to achieve, mourners feel a renewed sense of energy and confidence, an ability to fully acknowledge the reality of the death, and the capacity to become re-involved and reinvested in the activities of living. Working towards reconciliation means meeting the six needs of mourning, discussed later in this section.

Unique Influences on the Grief Experience

Obviously, the unique circumstances surrounding the catastrophic injury that leads to brain or cardiac death results in natural complications in grief and mourning. Beyond the unique circumstances of death, there are a multitude of additional factors that influence an individual's and family's response to death.

As you strive to bring sensitivity and compassion to your helping role, our hope is that the following discussion of factors that influence the grief journey will enhance your capacity to understand and support donor families. Following each factor are questions to ask yourself as you "companion" people to the best of your ability.

The Circumstances of the Death

Almost invariably, for organ donor families, brain death occurs following a sudden and unexpected injury. One or more of the following descriptions below may characterize the circumstances of the death for tissue and eye donor families as well. Whether alone or in combination, the circumstances of death can create natural complications as survivors do the work of mourning.

Sudden and unexpected death

When a death occurs suddenly and without warning, the family has no time to psychologically, emotionally, or spiritually prepare themselves for this new reality.

Premature and untimely death

The age of the person who died can impact the psychological acceptance of the death. The death of a child or someone who has been an active, previously healthy individual violates the assumptions we hold about the natural course of life. It is unnatural for a parent to bury a child or for someone in "the prime of life" to die suddenly and unexpectedly.

Avoidable or preventable death

When someone dies because of the direct consequences of another's negligence or self-inflicted injury, the death may be perceived as preventable. Survivors may experience prolonged, intense grief reactions when such deaths occur, often because they continue to blame themselves and feel a sense of culpability for the death or blame others and thus feel deep anger and resentment. For some, this sense of preventability evolves from unrealistic perceptions. For others, who may have actually contributed to the death, feelings of guilt and regret are particularly painful. A desire for vengeance or retaliation as well as interactions with the criminal justice system may also complicate the mourning process.

Stigmatized death

For donor families, stigmatized deaths may include suicide or homicide. When someone takes their own life or their life is taken from them by another human being, survivors may experience a multitude of emotions. Feelings of anger, despair, guilt, and shame are common. The many unanswered questions and lack of social support can often complicate the grief journey of families coping with a death by suicide or homicide.

Violent and traumatic death

The thoughts, images, and fears of a survivor whose loved one died a painful, violent death can naturally complicate the grief process. Feelings of fear and horror over the final moments of the person's life or seeing the mutilating injuries to the person's body can greatly impact coping. In addition, traumatic injuries can influence whether or not a family is able to view or have contact with the person's body.

The Nature of the Relationship with the Person Who Died

Different people will have their own unique responses to the same loss based on the relationship that existed between the person and the person who died. For example, with the death of a parent, observers will note that adult children will often grieve in totally different ways. This is only natural based on such influences as the prior attachment in the relationship and the function the relationship served for them. We know, for example, that relationships that have had strong components of ambivalence are more difficult to reconcile than those not as conflicted.

The Unique Characteristics of the Bereaved Person

Previous styles of responding to loss and other crises often are, to some extent, predictive of a person's response to the death of someone loved. If a person has always tried to keep herself distant or run away from crises, she may well follow this pattern when confronted with grief. Other personality factors such as self-esteem, values, and beliefs also have an impact on the bereaved person's unique response to grief. Any prior mental health problems are also influential.

The Unique Characteristics of the Person Who Died

What kind of person was the donor? Was he warm and caring or mean-spirited? Was he a good brother or father or son or was he irresponsible, uncommunicative, or distant? What role did he play in the family? Was he a stabilizing or a destructive influence? The answers to these questions will help you understand each bereaved family's unique loss.

The Family's Religious and Cultural Background

Different cultures are known for the various in which they express or repress their feelings. And different religious or spiritual orientations bring wildly varying understandings of death and its aftermath to the experience. Seek to understand how each donor family's religious and cultural background influences their unique grief journey. If you are unfamiliar with a certain culture's traditions or mores, ask the family or do some research on your own.

The Ritual or Funeral Experience

The donor family's grief journey will also be influenced by not only the donation experience and leave-taking ritual, but also the subsequent funeral or memorial ritual. Did a funeral or memorial service take place? Was it personalized and meaningful or was it generic and empty? A meaningful funeral can be an excellent way of helping initiate the six needs of mourning (see p. 110).

Questions to ask yourself as caregiver:

What were the unique circumstances surrounding the death?

How old was the person who died?

Was the death perceived as preventable?

Would this death be considered a "stigmatized" death?

Did a family member witness the death?

Did the family view or have contact with the body?

What was the person who died like?

What types of relationships did he have with the family in your care?

What are the unique bereaved individuals like?

What is this family's religious and cultural background?

Was there a leave-taking ritual?

What was the funeral or memorial ritual like for this family?

_____

_____

_____

_____

_____

_____

_____

_____

_____

_____

_____

_____

_____

_____

_____

Common Responses to Grief and "Companioning" Helping Roles

We have said that each person's grief is unique and that you must allow each donor family to teach you what their grief is like for them instead of the other way around. We have also said that there is no predictable order or timetable to grief.

Still, in your work with bereaved families, you will see many of the following grief responses. This does not mean that every family member will experience all of these feelings, nor does it mean that these are the "acceptable" feelings. This list is simply intended to provide you with a brief summary of the more common grief responses you will encounter in your work with donor families and suggested ways to facilitate the expression of these feelings.

Shock, denial, numbness, and disbelief

These feelings are nature's way of temporarily protecting the mourner from the reality of the death of someone loved. In reflecting on this experience, most mourners make comments like, "I was there, but yet I really wasn't." "It was like a dream." "I managed to do what needed to be done, but I didn't feel a part of it." "Somehow I made it through but I don't remember a lot of the details of it."

When no opportunity is available to anticipate a death, this constellation of feelings is typically heightened and prolonged. They act as an anesthetic; the pain is there, but the mourner does not experience it in its fullness. In a very real sense, the body and mind take over in an effort to help the person survive.

Typically a physiological component accompanies feelings of shock and numbness. Heart palpitations, queasiness, stomach pain, and dizziness are quite common. Hysterical crying, outbursts of anger, laughing, and even fainting are also frequently witnessed at this time.

Shock and numbness wane only at the pace mourners are able and ready to acknowledge feelings of loss. However, even after they become capable of embracing the reality of the loss, this dimension may resurface on birthdays, anniversary dates (particularly anniversary of the death), or when the family revisits a place that holds memories of the person who died.

CAREGIVER RESPONSE

In our experience, the primary task of the caregiver at this time is simply to "be with" the mourner. Quiet, caring, supportive companionship often becomes the person's greatest need. The art of being physically and emotionally present, while at the same time not invading the person's space, is not always an easy task. When we as helpers feel helpless, often our first inclination is to talk too much. Sit in sacred silence. Listen.

When at all possible, a quiet physical environment should be provided to the bereaved family. When in shock, people become more disoriented when bombarded with outside noise. Quiet can be comforting.

Disorganization, confusion, searching, and yearning

Often the most isolating and frightening part of the grief experience begins after the funeral. This is frequently when mourners begin to be confronted by the full reality of the death. This is when many people experience the "going crazy" syndrome. Mourners often feel restless, agitated, impatient, and confused. Disconnected thoughts may race through their minds and strong emotions overwhelm. They are unable to complete tasks. Time feels distorted. They feel like they're "going crazy."

A restless searching for the person who died is a common part of the experience. Yearning for the dead person and being preoccupied with memories lead to intense moments of distress.

Other common features during this time are difficulties with eating and sleeping. Many people experience loss of appetite while others overeat. Difficulty in going to sleep and early morning awakenings are also common.

CAREGIVER RESPONSE

During this complex dimension of grief, the mourner tends to worry about the normalcy of her experience. She is not only faced with the pain of grief but also the fear that she may be "going crazy." You can offer reassurance and education about the normalcy of the experience. You can also help by listening to the mourner's story. Be patient and attentive, even if the family tells the same stories over and over or needs to talk and cry for long periods of time. The role of the helper is not to interrupt with reasoning, but to be present and empathetic.

Anxiety, panic, and fear

Feelings of anxiety, panic, and fear are often experienced by mourners. These feelings are typically generated from thoughts such as, "Will my life have any purpose without this person? I don't think I can live without him."

As the person's mind is continually brought back to the pain of loss, panic may set in. Fear of what the future holds; fear that one person's death will result in others; fear that the donation recipient(s) will die, too, increased awareness of one's own mortality; feelings of vulnerability about being able to survive without the person; inability to concentrate; and emotional and physical fatigue all serve to heighten anxiety, panic, and fear. The mourner often feels overwhelmed by everyday problems and concerns. To make matters worse, a change in financial security may have resulted from the death; large bills may need to be paid and the fear of becoming dependent on others often increases, as well.

CAREGIVER RESPONSE

While mourners will often talk about their feelings of loss, they are less likely to bring up the topic of their fears. Fears sometimes seem silly or weak in a way that other emotions do not. You can help by asking open-ended questions such as, "Other donor families have taught me that the death has brought about fears. Have you had feelings of fear since the death?" This will provide the family with an opportunity to explore these difficult feelings.

Physiological changes

At a time of acute grief, a person's body responds to what the mind has been told. Some of the most common physiological changes that the mourner may experience are as follows:

- generalized lack of energy and fatigue
- shortness of breath
- feelings of emptiness in the stomach
- tightness in the throat and chest
- sensitivity to noise
- heart palpitations
- queasiness
- difficulty in sleeping or sometimes prolonged sleeping
- headaches
- agitation and generalized tension

With loss, the mourner's immune system breaks down and he or she becomes vulnerable to illness. In fact, many studies have documented significant increases in illness following bereavement. In the majority of cases, however, physical symptoms are normal and temporary.

CAREGIVER RESPONSE

Be aware that physical disorders prior to the loss tend to become worse after the loss. Transient identification with the cause of death is also common. For example, if a husband suffered an aneurysm and was later declared brain dead, the wife may begin to complain of headaches.

Depending on the extent of the symptoms, suggesting that the mourner consult a physician is appropriate to rule out physical causes. A general exam often helps reassure the mourner that he is well and needn't be overly concerned about his physical health.

Explosive emotions

The explosive emotions of grief—including anger, hate, blame, resentment, rage, and jealousy—are very common among survivors of a sudden and violent death. It is natural for family members to be angry that someone they loved was taken from them so unexpectedly and so brutally. They may be angry at those they hold responsible for the death, at God, or at themselves. Sometimes family members are angry at each other over a perceived lack of support, selfishness, or disengagement.

Because of our society's attitude toward anger, explosive emotions are often the most upsetting to those around the mourner. We often simply don't know how to respond to anger. Yet anger in grief serves a healthy purpose: It helps mourners temporarily protest the painful reality of the loss. It's as if having the capacity to express anger gives one the courage to survive at this moment in time. The mourner who does not give herself permission to be angry, if she is, or whose feelings of anger are squelched or frowned upon by others, may slide into chronic depression.

CAREGIVER RESPONSE

As always, you can help the angry mourner realize that her feelings are normal and necessary. Many grieving people need a supportive listener who can tolerate, encourage, and validate explosive emotions without judging, retaliating, or arguing.

You can also make suggestions for appropriate outlets of expression. Physical activities such as walking, jogging, biking, and swimming are good ways to release explosive emotions. Less active ways include journaling, writing a letter to the person the mourner is angry with (but perhaps not mailing it), and painting or other artwork.

Guilt and remorse

Guilt and self-blame are also very common responses to a sudden and violent death. If a death was caused by an accident or was self-inflicted, it is often perceived as preventable. "If only I would have. . ." and "Why didn't I . . ." are two typical thought patterns among family members. "Why wasn't I the one to die?" is yet another guilty feeling.

Guilt can also be experienced when the mourner begins to re-experience any kind of joy or happiness in his life. This often relates to loyalty to the person who died and fears that being happy in some way betrays the relationship that once was.

You will also witness occasions when feelings of guilt will be induced by others. This often occurs through ignorance, lack of understanding, or the need to project one's own feelings outside one's self. Projecting is illustrated by family members who, in wanting to deny their own pain and any sense of culpability, strike out against other family members.

CAREGIVER RESPONSE

As caregivers, we often want to unburden survivor families of their feelings of guilt and remorse. "But it wasn't your fault!" we might say to them. "You're not to blame!" While these statements may be true, offering them too early in our conversations with the bereaved family prevents family members from expressing these normal and necessary feelings. Try to avoid the urge to quickly and prematurely explain the person's guilt away. Only in exploring what he should or should not feel guilty about—and deciding for himself—does the mourner come to some peace with what the limits of his responsibility are.

We must acknowledge that guilt can be, and often is for donor families, a component of complicated grief, particularly chronic depression, and cannot be ignored. Guilt is one of the most frequent emotional realms in which people become trapped and have difficulties. Perhaps you could facilitate a discussion among family members to help express and reconcile bottled-up thoughts and feelings of guilt and blame.

Loss, emptiness, and sadness

With good reason, this constellation of feelings and experiences is often the most difficult for the mourner. As we have said, the full sense of the loss never occurs all at once. Months often pass before mourners are confronted by how much their lives have changed.

In our work with thousands of mourners, we have learned that they struggle most with feelings of loss, emptiness, and sadness at the following times: weekends; holidays; upon waking up in the morning; late at night, particularly at bedtime; family meal times; upon arriving home to an empty house; and any kind of birthday or anniversary occasion.

Unfortunately, many people surrounding the mourners frequently try to take these feelings away. Friends, family, and sometimes even professional caregivers erroneously believe that their job is to distract the mourner from these feelings.

CAREGIVER RESPONSE

Because this dimension of grief is so isolating, the opportunity to communicate one's feelings to an accepting and understanding person is one means of reconnecting with the world outside oneself. One goal of helping is to keep the person from feeling totally isolated and abandoned during this difficult time. Many people respond to an outreach approach, as the sense of isolation may prevent them from asking directly for support and guidance.

To counteract society's tendency to discourage the expression of these feelings, the mourner needs to be encouraged to share thoughts and express tears. You can provide a "safe place" for the expression of painful emotions. You can help the mourner understand that these feelings and these tears are not shameful or signs of weakness but indeed signs of strength and healing.

The Six Reconciliation Needs of Mourning

The death of someone loved changes our lives forever. And the movement from the "before" to the "after" is almost always a long, painful journey. From our own experiences with loss as well as those of the thousands of grieving people we have worked with over the years, we have learned that if we are to heal, we cannot skirt the outside edges of our grief. Instead, we must journey all through it, sometimes meandering the side roads, sometimes plowing directly into its raw center.

There are six "yield signs" donor families are likely to encounter on their journey through grief—what we call the "reconciliation needs of mourning." For while their grief journeys will be intensely personal, unique experiences, all mourners must yield to this set of basic human needs if they are to heal.

Grief or Clinical Depression?

You may wonder when feelings of loss, emptiness, and sadness are intense enough to be considered depression. Following are guidelines that may help you make this distinction.

Grief	Clinical Depression
Responds to comfort and support	Does not accept support
Often openly angry	Irritable and may complain but does not directly express anger
Relates depressed feelings to loss to a particular event	Does not relate feelings
Can still experience moments of enjoyment in life	Exhibits an all-pervading sense of doom
May have transient physical complaints	Has chronic physical complaints
Expresses guilt over some specific aspect of the loss	Has generalized feelings of guilt
Has temporary impact on self-esteem	Presents a deep loss of esteem

Of course, suicidal thoughts or actions are also red-flag behaviors and should be taken seriously. Many mourners do have transient thoughts of suicide, wishing to be reunited with the person who died or simply to escape the pain of grief. While such thoughts are normal, they must always be explored and followed with the utmost care.

Earlier in this resource we briefly addresses Needs 1 & 2. Here we reiterate them and explore the remaining needs of mourning.

Need 1. Acknowledging the reality of the death.

This first need of mourning involves gently confronting the reality that someone the mourner cared about will never physically come back into her life again.

Especially in cases where the death was sudden, acknowledging the full reality of the loss may occur over months and even years. To survive, she may try to push away the reality of the death at times. She may discover herself replaying events surrounding the death and confronting memories, both good and bad. This replay is a vital part of this need of mourning. It's as if each time she talks it out, the event is a little more real.

Remember—this first need of mourning, like the other five that follow, may intermittently require her attention for months, sometimes years. As a caregiver, you must be patient and compassionate as donor family members work on each of them.

Need 2. Embracing the pain of the loss.

This need of mourning requires mourners to embrace the pain of the loss—something they naturally don't want to do. It is easier to avoid, repress, or deny the pain of grief than it is to confront it, yet it is in confronting pain that we learn to reconcile ourselves to it.

You will probably discover that mourners need to "dose" themselves in embracing their pain. In other words, they cannot (nor should they try to) overload themselves with the hurt all at once. Sometimes they may need to distract themselves from the pain of death, while at other times you will need to help them create a safe place to move toward it.

Unfortunately, our culture tends to encourage the denial of pain. If mourners openly express their feelings of grief, misinformed friends may advise them to "carry on" or "keep your chin up." If, on the other hand, they remain "strong" and "in control," they may be congratulated for "doing well" with their grief. Actually, doing well with their grief means becoming well acquainted with their pain.

Need 3. Remembering the person who died.

Do you have any kind of relationship with someone when they die? Of course. You have a relationship of memory. Precious memories, dreams reflecting the significance of the relationship, and objects that link you to the person who died (such as photos, souvenirs etc.) are examples of some of the things that give testimony to a different form of a continued relationship. This need of mourning involves allowing and encouraging mourners to pursue this relationship.

But some people may try to take mourners' memories away. Trying to be helpful, they encourage them to take down all the photos of the person who died. They tell them to keep busy or even to move out of their house. But in our experience, remembering the past makes hoping for the future possible. Their future will become open to new experiences only to the extent that they embrace the past.

Need 4. Developing a new self-identity.

Part of your self-identity comes from the relationships you have with other people. When someone with whom you have a relationship dies, your self-identity, or the way you see yourself, naturally changes.

Bereaved spouses may go from being a "wife" or "husband" to a "widow" or "widower." Others may have go from being a "parent" to a "bereaved parent." The way they define themselves and the way society defines them is changed.

A death often requires family members to take on new roles that had been filled by the person who died. After all, someone still has to take out the garbage, someone still has to buy the groceries. Mourners confront their changed identity every time they do something that used to be done by the person who died. This can be very hard work and can leave them feeling very drained.

Mourners may occasionally feel child-like as they struggle with their changing identities. They may feel a temporarily heightened dependence on others as well as feelings of helplessness, frustration, inadequacy, and fear.

Many donor family members discover that as they work on this need, they ultimately discover some positive aspects of their changed self-identities. They may develop a renewed confidence in themselves, for example. Through the donation experience, they often find a more caring, kind, and sensitive part of themselves. They may develop an assertive part of their identity that empowers them to go on living even though they continue to feel a sense of loss.

Need 5. Searching for meaning.

When someone loved dies, survivors naturally question the meaning and purpose of life. They often question their philosophy of life and explore religious and spiritual values as they work on this need. They may discover themselves searching for meaning in their continued living as they ask "How?" and "Why" questions.

"How could God let this happen?" "Why did this happen now, in this way?" The death reminds them of their lack of control. It can leave them feeling powerless.

The person who died was a part of each donor family member. This death means they mourn a loss not only outside of themselves, but inside of themselves as well. At times, overwhelming sadness and loneliness may be their constant companions. Survivors often say that when this person died, part of them died, too. And now they are faced with finding some meaning in going on with their lives— even though they feel so empty.

This death also calls for survivors to confront their own spirituality. They may doubt their faith and have spiritual conflicts and questions racing through their head and heart. This is normal and part of their journey toward renewed living.

Need 6. Receiving ongoing support from others.

The quality and quantity of understanding support survivors get during their grief journey will have a major influence on their capacity to heal. They cannot—nor should they try to—do this alone. You can help them see that drawing on the experiences and encouragement of friends, fellow mourners, or professional counselors is not a weakness but a healthy human need. And because mourning is a process that takes place over time, this support must be available months and even years after the death.

Unfortunately, because our society places so much value on the ability to "carry on," "keep your chin up" and "keep busy," many mourners are abandoned shortly after the event of the death. "It's over and done with" and "It's time to get on with your life" are the types of messages directed at mourners that still dominate. Obviously, these messages encourage the denial and repression of grief rather than its expression.

To be truly helpful, the people in the mourner's support system— including you as caregiver—must appreciate the impact this death has had on the family. They must understand that in order to heal, family members must be allowed—even encouraged—to mourn long after the death. And they must encourage them to see mourning not as an enemy to be vanquished but as a necessity to be experienced as a result of having loved.

The Special Needs of Grieving Children

Adults grieve. So do children. In fact, anyone old enough to love is old enough to grieve. Even before children are able to talk, they grieve when someone loved dies. And these feelings about the death become a part of their lives forever.

Caring adults can help children during this time. If adults are open, honest, and loving, experiencing the loss of someone loved can be a chance for children to learn about both the joy and the pain that comes from caring deeply for other people.

- *Be a good observer. See how each child is behaving. Don't rush in with explanations. Usually it's more helpful to ask exploring questions than to give quick answers.*

- *Don't expect children's reactions to be obvious and immediate. Be patient and be available. Children often grieve more through behaviors than words, and they tend to grieve in "doses," allowing in just a little of the reality at a time.*

- *Children are part of the family, too. And reassurance comes from the presence of loving people. Children feel secure in the care of gentle arms and tenderness.*

- *Use simple, direct language with children when talking about the death. Don't use euphemisms.*

- *Be honest about the death and the donation, using child-friendly language when you communicate.*

- *Allow children to express a full range of feelings. Anger, guilt, despair, and protest are natural reactions to the death of someone loved.*

Caring for Donor Families

Reconciling Grief

Sometimes people will come to you with the expectation that their grief will end when they resolve, or recover from, their grief. But their grief journeys will never end. People do not "get over" grief.

Reconciliation is a term we find more appropriate for what occurs as the mourner works to integrate the new reality of moving forward in life without the physical presence of the person who died. With reconciliation comes a renewed sense of energy and confidence, an ability to fully acknowledge the reality of the death, and a capacity to become reinvolved and reinvested in the activities of living.

In reconciliation, the sharp, ever-present pain of grief gives rise to a renewed sense of meaning and purpose. Feelings of loss will not completely disappear, yet they will soften, and the intense pangs of grief will become less frequent. Hope for a continued life will emerge as family members are able to make commitments to the future, realizing that the person who died will never be forgotten, yet knowing that their lives can and will move forward.

Please note that while we use the term "healing" in grief throughout this text, we do not use it in the traditional medical sense of the word. To be bereaved is to be torn apart and forever changed. Yes, healing and reconciliation do emerge (if the mourner's needs are met and their grief expressed), but mourners are never "all better" or "back to normal." They have learned to integrate the loss into their lives—perhaps even to better their lives as a result of the loss—but the profound pain and sadness inherent in loss never fully subside. Grief is a never-ending, lifelong process.

Seven Central Helping Roles for Bereavement Caregivers

1. *Listening to the bereaved.*
   Empathetic listening is an essential helping principle. To listen effectively means that the caregiver does not have all of the answers and needs the communication of the mourner as a guide to know how to respond in helpful ways. The mourner feels validated when he is heard. Empathetic listening allows the caregiver to "be with" the mourner, encouraging the expression of grief and the telling of the story.

2. *Understanding the bereaved*
   To understand the bereaved means to be familiar with thoughts, feelings, and behaviors common to the grief experience. Beyond understanding is the task of communicating this understanding back to the bereaved in a helpful way. This capacity to understand and then check perception is best achieved by caregivers who adopt a "teach me" attitude.

3. *Educating the bereaved*
   While the bereaved donor family must be your teacher about their unique grief experience, it is your role to affirm the normalcy and naturalness of their thoughts and feelings. Many newly bereaved people are not familiar with what is normal in grief, particularly when they have no prior experience with loss. It's important to help mourners know that they aren't "going crazy," for example, as they experience the common disorientation and anxieties of grief.

4. *Supporting the bereaved*
   The process of supporting the bereaved follows naturally from educating. To support means to accompany mourners on the journey through the healthy reconciliation of grief. The caregiver's supportive counseling skills provide structure and validation for the expression of grief and a safe place for donor families to do the work of mourning.

5. *Advocating for the bereaved*
   Caregivers must advocate for donor families. During the donation process, this may mean supporting the family's need to spend more time with the body and helping ensure that a leavetaking ritual takes place. After the donation, this may mean making sure donor families have the information they seek (and are allowed to have) about organ and tissue recipients or other concerns and questions.

6. *Encouraging the bereaved*
   The encouraging caregiver projects a hopefulness about the mourner's capacity to achieve reconciliation. Encouraging is

Caring for Donor Families

*a process of assisting mourners in restoring a sense of self,
establishing new relationships and activities, and going on with
life while at the same time acknowledging that a significant loss
has occurred.*

7. *Referring the bereaved*
    *Referring the bereaved is a necessary skill for all caregivers.
    Appropriate referral means the caregiver must be aware of his
    or her own level of counseling skills and, when necessary, must
    skillfully facilitate the transfer of care to a more qualified
    helper. Some complicated grief responses require specialized
    interventions and additional training.*

Development of a Family Support Project: A Working Model

"Organ donation is a phenomenon, not a transaction." Recently, one donor mother used these words to describe her thoughts following her son's donation. With these words she teaches us that donation is much more than simply an act of giving, or a set of procedures to procure and place organs. Donation is a lifelong companion to the grief a family will experience.

Just as bereaved individuals do not "get over" grief, a donor family does not forget that donation took place. The organ or tissue recovery is not the end of the "donation process" for these families. It is the beginning of a lifelong journey. The fact that a family chooses donation, experiences the donation process, and provides a gift to others creates special issues during their grief journey as they do the work of mourning. These issues create special needs, including the need for ongoing support.

Developing an aftercare program for donor families is a natural extension of the care provided to them before and during their donation experience. What does your organization offer bereaved donor families in the months and years following their family member's death and donation?

For many individuals and agencies, the most difficult step is deciding where to begin. What follows is a working model for developing a donor family support program that meets the unique needs of your families as well as the needs of your organization. Several phases for program development are outlined below. A brief description of each phase is followed by a series of questions designed to guide you as you determine the most appropriate services to offer families in your area.

Phase One—Determining Families' Needs

The immediate as well as the long-term needs of survivors are diverse and ever-changing. In your desire to develop a successful program, you must begin by exploring not only the needs of donor families in your area but the needs of your organization and community, as well. You may find it helpful to develop a needs assessment survey, sponsor an open forum, or host a focus group during your initial phase of information gathering. Invite donor family members, procurement staff, hospital representatives, hospice or funeral home staff, representatives of local grief support groups, and members of other agencies offering aftercare in your area. Donor families have much to contribute to this process from the beginning. When possible, involve donor families early on in your planning and establishment of the program. Communicate about the type of support that is already available to bereaved families (there are probably few services directly aimed at meeting the unique needs of donor families) and determine the voids that your agency might fill. With an awareness of the characteristics of the families you hope to support (survivors of sudden death, suicide and homicide survivors, bereaved parents, siblings, children, etc.) you may begin to formulate some ideas about the types of services that donor families may find beneficial.

Questions to ask yourself as caregiver:

What bereavement aftercare services are already offered in your community?

Are their special services only your agency can offer donor families?

How much is your organization willing and able to invest in aftercare?

_____

_____

_____

_____

_____

_____

Consider This

Consider who is in need of your support services. Will your agency be providing support to only the donor's "legal next of kin?" Will you provide services for children and adolescents in the family? Are your support services available to all donor families regardless of what was donated (e.g., organs, tissues or eyes, aborted donor cases, and non-donor families)?

Consider the type of record-keeping system that will be necessary for accessing information about families receiving support. When the aftercare provider is communicating with a family by telephone, will the following important information be easily accessible: the family member's relationship to the person who died, nature of the death, date of death, age, gender and ethnicity of the donor, recipient information, names of staff who cared for the family during the donation process, etc.? With each contact a family should feel that your care for them continues. Care did not end when they completed the donation consent forms and left the hospital.

Conveying to a family that you are aware of the circumstances of their family member's death (e.g., how long it has been since the death) or that you remember the name of the person who died offers reassurance to a family that they are important to your agency and that their gift has not been forgotten.

Phase Two—Establishing a Vision

Once donor family, organizational, and community needs are determined, you will be ready to establish a vision for your agency's aftercare program. Outlining the purpose of your program through a mission statement and creating specific goals will help you determine the types of services that should be offered to families in your area.

Take a moment to draft a preliminary vision statement for your agency. Use your imagination. Be creative. Write it in the form of a mission, program objectives, or a list of the services you believe families would find invaluable.

My Vision Statement

_____
_____
_____
_____
_____
_____
_____
_____

Initially, your agency may be reluctant to provide support beyond supplying information concerning the donation to families. There may be concern that the staff is not "qualified" to provide support to a family as they continue their grief journey. We remind you of your role as "companion" to these families. During this difficult life transition, family members are searching for someone who will listen, not advise. Someone who will validate the humanness in their pain, not try to take the pain away. Caregivers from your agencies have already demonstrated this level of caring before and during the donation experience. Certainly those designated to care for families after the donation should exhibit the capacity to "companion" bereaved donor family members as well. By offering compassionate ongoing support, your agency has the unique opportunity to give voice to each family's grief and donation experience rather than silencing it.

Aftercare coordinators are given a unique opportunity to actively participate in the family's journey. Allow yourself to learn from each family's unique experience. There is no need to feel you have to be the "expert" on grief and donation to provide good aftercare. Instead, be available, listen, and offer supportive presence as they embrace the painful loss of someone loved.

As you "companion" families, your primary support goals may include providing opportunities for affiliation, understanding grief, normalizing their experience, providing emotional support, offering access to community resources, educating staff about grief and loss, etc. Once you've outlined primary goals, you must choose how you will provide these support services. For example, emotional support may be provided to families through phone calls, online through the internet, or home visits following the funeral ceremony. Offer only services that you can realistically provide to families and be prepared to follow through on promises made.

Questions to ask yourself as caregiver:

Has your agency established a vision of the services that will be offered to families?

Have you taken time to develop a mission statement that will guide the care being provided?

Are the services you will offer practical and based on the needs of the families in your area?

What is your primary role with each family (e.g., advocate, counselor, informant, etc.)?

What type of additional training will assist you in offering the best care to families?

_____

_____

_____

_____

_____

_____

_____

_____

Selecting an Aftercare Coordinator

An important element to developing a successful family support program is selecting the right person to coordinate it. Who is "qualified" to offer this type of care to donor families? While knowledge and skills in the area of counseling and bereavement are important, recognize that differences in training do exist across fields. Social workers, master-level counselors, family therapists, nurses, chaplains, and others all have vastly divergent training experiences. Training in clinical helping skills is essential in offering support in person as well as over the telephone. Degrees can be deceiving; be sure to inquire about clinical experiences during the interview process.

Looking beyond education, a multitude of personal qualities should also be considered (e.g., compassion, empathy, and genuineness). Below are several questions that may assist you in your search for the right person to coordinator your agency's program.

- *What is this person's philosophy on helping bereaved families?*

- *Will this person be attentive and responsive to families' needs?*

- *Does this person have the capacity to be fully present as he or she interacts with families?*

- *Are his or her basic helping skills proficient (e.g., listening, empathy, and summarizing)?*

Phase Three—Developing The Program

With your vision and goals in mind (and on paper), the next step is to develop a blueprint for your program. This will involve determining the dimensions and content of communication with families. The dimensions of communication will include deciding how support will be offered (e.g., in-person, by telephone, mail, e-mail, internet chat rooms, or support groups). If you've gathered information from other aftercare agencies, you may want to reference the content of communications sent to families as you begin to create your own letters, cards, and pamphlets.

Additionally, your blueprint will illustrate how frequently and for what length of time your agency will be in contact with families. Perhaps the aftercare coordinator will initiate contact monthly, every three months, or twice a year. There are no rules as to how long your agency should provide this level of support to families. Your aftercare program may be as brief as six months or contact may continue for several years.

Here we offer an illustration of an 18-month follow-up program designed in 1998 to meet the needs of donor families in the state of Iowa. As described above, this program was created from an amalgamation of resources gathered both locally and nationally. As all programs should, this aftercare program is continuously being modified to meet the changing needs of donor families as well as accommodate the tremendous growth within the agency since its initial development.

In addition to scheduled mailings or contacts with families, you may choose to offer additional support by providing opportunities for families to remember and share their story about the person who died. This may be in the form of memorial projects such as quilts, a memorial garden, or a book honoring donor family stories. Perhaps your agency will host a ceremony to recognize and commemorate the person who died. Tree planting dedications and holiday remembrance ceremonies are just two ways in which

Family Follow-Up Sample Form

Donor Name: _____ Age/Sex/Race: _____

Hospital: _____ OPC: _____

Date of Death: _____ Cause of Death: _____

Recipients:

Heart: _____ Liver: _____ Lungs: _____ Kidneys: _____

Pancreas: _____ Small Intestine: _____ Bone ____ Skin ____ Heart Valves ____ Eyes ____

Family Information:

Family Name: _____ Relationship: _____

Address: _____ Phone: _____

TYPE OF CONTACT	DATE	COORDINATOR
Initial Contact by Donation/Procurement Coordinator (immediately following the donation, check the following) ___ Phone Call made to family ___ Family did not wish to be called		
Billing Information Letter (Informs families of whom to call with billing questions and concerns)		
Initial Letter containing recipient information (send within 2 weeks following the death and donation) • Include business card of Aftercare Coordinator • Information on writing to recipients (anonymously)		
Follow-up Call (after family has received billing information and initial receipt information letter) ___ Made by the Aftercare Coordinator		
1 Month: *Afterwords* Grief Packet • Include inserts regarding special local projects such as Memory Tree, Donor Family Quilt • Include *Understanding brain death: A simple explanation* • Include other relevant inserts specific to the type of death (suicide, homicide, death of a child)		
3 Month: Need Assessment Survey (Provides families opportunity to reflect on their experience and the option to continue to receive follow-up)		
6 Month: Letter (and telephone contact when possible) • Include list of recommended books on grief and/or donation or list of books in your lending library and local/national support group resource list • Include *To Give & Grieve* book and copy of National Donor Family Council Newsletter		
9 Month: Letter to Family with Butterfly Donor Family Pin		
1 Year: card during the week Anniversary of the death		
15 Month: Thinking of you Note or Card		
18 Month: Letter and Needs Assessment Survey (Informs families of the activities they will continue to be informed of until they wish to no longer have contact with the procurement agency)		
Note: A book on coping during the holidays is sent during the first holiday season following the death.		

you can remind families that their precious family member and the gift they shared will be remembered always.

Directing the family toward useful donation and bereavement resources may be an important ingredient in your aftercare. Materials on grief and donation can be made available through a lending library. A list of local support groups can be procured and distributed to families. You have a wonderful opportunity to assist families in finding a variety of support resources. Help them to reach out beyond your agency for assistance during this difficult time, and find support with others within their community and nationally as well. As difficult as it may be, because of the tendency for us to be protective of "our families," it will be necessary for you to allow them to continue their growth and extend their circles of support on their own.

Consider developing a newsletter that focuses on issues specific to bereaved donor families. Offer information on national support services (e.g., National Kidney Foundation Donor Family Council and Compassionate Friends). Provide opportunities for families to affiliate with other donor families as well as transplant recipients through support groups, workshops, picnics, and other events. Consider developing a bereavement volunteer program to facilitate the process of families supporting families during or after their donation experience. Donor families often participate in these special events long after their loss.

You may be supporting a family that does not live in your area because they did not live close to the person who died or the person who died did not reside locally. These families often find comfort in being informed of the support and events available in their area as well. Collaborate with the procurement agencies, funeral homes, and hospices in the area to develop a list of contacts and resources for these families.

Questions to ask yourself as caregiver:

What services do we want to provide to families?

How long do we want our program to be?

_____

_____

_____

_____

_____

_____

_____

_____

_____

Phase Four—Selecting Resources and Materials

Careful consideration should be made when selecting resources and materials for your program. Materials should be compatible with the designated needs and established goals of your program. A number of bereavement and donation resources exist (see the list of national resources on p. 153). Consider resources that provide new knowledge but also review information you assume that families were already told during their hospital experience. For example, you may offer information concerning brain death and guidelines for anonymous communication with transplant recipients. The initial letters to the family may remind the family to contact the procurement agency with any billing concerns.

When selecting materials, take time to examine information offered by hospices, hospitals, funeral homes, and procurement agencies in your area. Seek recommendations from staff and whenever possible, donor families themselves. Other considerations to make when selecting materials include cost and storage capacity.

Supporting Donor Families in an Era of Long-Distance Communication

We recognize that it is not always feasible for you as an aftercare coordinator to engage in person-to-person follow-up care with donor families. Indeed, a good portion of your contact with families may be by letter, telephone, or internet (e-mail or chat rooms). These forms of communication may not be the ideal mode of facilitating ongoing support to families, but this is the reality for many agencies servicing a large geographic area.

Remember, the distance between you and the family need not prevent you from developing and maintaining an authentic relationship with them. Indeed, offering emotional support and information, conveying understanding and empathy, and interpreting responses over the telephone or by e-mail can be challenging. Below we offer a few practical ideas for offering support to families wherever they may be.

- *Familiarize yourself with the family's story. Invite caregivers who are familiar with the family's experience to share their thoughts on offering continued support to them.*

- *Be aware of your surroundings and create a space that will facilitate the helping process. Seek out a quiet, private area free of distractions and interruptions, where you feel able to communicate openly, candidly, and sensitively with family members.*

- *Soften your jumpstart. Within the first moments of contact, you set the tone for this and future communications you will have with the family. As you introduce yourself, your role, and the reason for your call, letter, or online contact, convey to the family that you are familiar with their experience and, more important, that you care how they are feeling now, after the death and donation.*

- *If making a phone call, inquire about the appropriateness of your timing in making this contact. This is particularly important in situations where the family is not anticipating your call.*

- *Communicate genuine respect, empathy, acceptance, and non-judgment as the family shares personal, and at times intense, feelings, concerns, fears, or questions with you.*

- *Listen attentively, ensuring the person knows you are "with" them and interested in what they are sharing. Identify feelings and check the accuracy of your perceptions as you communicate with the family ("It sounds like..." "What I hear you saying is...").*

- *Use this time to address whatever the family is teaching you about their needs at this time, including practical as well as emotional needs.*

- *Following your contact, take a few minutes to document the exchange, recording enough information to remind you of the important pieces of this conversation the next time you connect with the family.*

Questions to ask yourself as caregiver:

Would you prefer to purchase professionally produced materials or create your own?

Are the materials you've selected outdated or do they contain inaccurate information?

Are the materials sensitive to the diverse cultural beliefs and values of families?

_____

_____

_____

_____

_____

_____

_____

_____

_____

_____

Affiliating with Other Donor Families: A Key to Aftercare

Grief can be an isolating experience. Donating the organs or tissues of a family member may add to the feelings of alienation and isolation a family feels. Families have shared with us that even when they find others who've experienced a loss similar to their own, they are unable to share special feelings and ponder questions related to the donation. An important part of the donor family's grief journey may include exploring questions related to the giving of the gift with others who, like them, made the decision to help others through donation. A husband may find comfort knowing that somewhere in the world his wife's heart is still beating. A mother may experience concern over a young recipient's health. Feelings of deep sadness may be felt once again upon hearing of a recipient's death. There is an inherent curiosity about the recipient, and many families wonder if they will ever have the chance to meet the person who lives on because of their decision to donate.

Phase Five—Program Implementation and Evaluation

Now that you have established the purpose, developed a blueprint, and selected resource materials for your agency's program, it is time to open your doors and invite the families in. The program coordinator should be prepared for an influx of calls. Now that you've anticipated the unmet needs of families and are reaching out to families (that's right, you are no longer waiting for them to contact you first), be ready for families to reach back.

At the same time, it is important to remember to respect a family's right to decline your services. The frequency of contact may not suit all families, and not every family will desire the materials you've chosen. Be certain to allow families the opportunity within the first few months of contact to "opt out" or to continue participation in the aftercare provided. This may be as simple as including information on how to discontinue participation in a letter sent a few months following the death.

A valuable aftercare program is one that families find beneficial and one that adapts to their changing needs. Whenever possible, create opportunities for families to guide program modifications or devise new projects. Ask active family members to review new letters, surveys, or project ideas before they are offered. Listen to their recommendations. Utilize tools such as surveys, family forums, retreats, or workshops to provide opportunities for donor families to comment on the quality and appropriateness of your services. At the same time, special events such as these will provide families with the freedom to acknowledge and explore openly, with one another, what it means to grieve as a donor family.

Questions to ask yourself as caregiver:

What opportunities will be made available to families to evaluate or offer suggestions on your agency's aftercare services?

What type of additional follow-up will be given to families who share dissatisfaction with the donation experience?

Does your family support project offer opportunities for families to affiliate and connect with one another or with transplant recipients?

_____

_____

_____

_____

_____

_____

_____

_____

_____

_____

Incorporating Self-Care for the Caregiver into Your Program

For caregivers to the bereaved, good self-care is critical for at least three major reasons. First and most important, we owe it to ourselves and our families to lead joyful, whole lives. While caring for donor families is certainly rewarding, we cannot and should not expect our work to fulfill us completely.

Second, our work is draining—physically, emotionally, and spiritually. Assisting bereaved people is a demanding interpersonal process that requires much energy and focus. Whenever we attempt to respond to the needs of those in grief, chances are slim that we can (or should) avoid the stress of emotional involvement. Each day we open ourselves to caring about donor families and their personal life journeys. And genuinely caring about people touches the depths of our hearts and souls. We need respite from such draining work.

And third, we owe it to donor families themselves. Our personal experience and observation suggest that good self-care is an essential foundation of caring for and meaningfully companioning the bereaved. They are sensitive to our ability to "be with" them. Poor self-care results in distraction from the helping relationship, and bereaved people often intuit when we are not physically, emotionally, and spiritually available to them.

Poor self-care can also cause caregivers to distance themselves from people's pain by trying to act like an expert. Because many of us have been trained to remain professionally distant, we may stay aloof from the very people we are supposed to help. Generally, this is a projection of our own need to stay distant from the pain of others, as well as from our own life hurts. The "expert mode" is antithetical to compassionate care and can cause an irreparable rift between you and donor families.

So, does this work have to be exhausting? Naturally draining, yes, but exhausting? We don't think so. Good helpers naturally focus outward, resulting in a drain on both head and heart! Of course, you will hear some people say, "If you do this kind of caregiving, you might as well resign yourself to eventually burning out." Again, we don't think so. The key is to practice daily, ongoing, nurturing self-care. To do so, you may need to try on some new ways of thinking and being.

The Bereavement Caregiver's Self-Care Guidelines

The following self-care guidelines are not intended to be cure-alls, nor will they be appropriate for everyone. Pick and choose those tips that you believe will be of help to you in your efforts to stay physically and emotionally healthy.

Remember, our attitudes about stress and fatigue in general sometimes make it difficult to make changes. However, one important point to remember is that with support and encouragement from others, most of us can learn to make positive changes in our attitudes and behaviors.

You might find it helpful to have a discussion among coworkers about caregiver fatigue syndrome. Identify your own signs and symptoms of burnout. Discuss individual and group approaches to self-care that will help you enjoy both work and play.

The Joy of Mini-Vacations

What creative ideas can you come up with to renew yourself? Caregivers are notorious for helping others create self-care time while neglecting their own needs. Here are a few ideas to get you started. However, I encourage you to create your own list and pursue them.

- Schedule a massage with a professional massage therapist
- Have a spiritual growth weekend. Retreat into nature. Plan some alone time.
- Go for a drive with no particular destination in mind. Explore the countryside, slow down, and observe what you see.
- Treat yourself to a night in a hotel or bed and breakfast.
- Visit a museum or a zoo.
- Go for a hot air balloon ride.
- Take an afternoon off and go to the movies—maybe even a kid's movie!
- Go to a yard sale or auction.
- Go rollerskating or rollerblading with a friend!
- Enjoy a photographic retreat. Take your camera into nature and shoot away.
- Watch cartoons with a child.
- Visit a farmer's market and shop for fresh produce.
- Drop by a health food store and walk the aisles.
- Go dancing.
- Take a horseback ride.
- Plan a river-rafting trip.

What ideas can you come up with?

_____

_____

_____

_____

_____

Remember Your Child-Like Self

Have you ever met the overly-serious caregiver who projects gloom and doom? Odds are she has forgotten the vitality and enthusiasm of her childhood years. Let's pause and recall some of the characteristics of childhood.

Children:

- *are physically connected to the world around them.*
- *take risks.*
- *are open, enthusiastic learners.*
- *imagine and dream.*
- *are naturally curious.*
- *spontaneously laugh and smile a lot.*
- *are passionate and expressive.*
- *try new things when they get bored.*
- *rest when they need rest.*
- *try to have fun whenever they can.*

So, have you "grown up" and forgotten about the joy of being a child? If so, you may have left behind some of the best self-care strategies ever. Think about the way healthy kids go about their day, then think about how you spend your day. Have you forgotten how vital fun is to life and living?

There is a well-established link between play and energy. Play should be a vital part of your self-care plan. Being grown-up doesn't mean always being serious. Most really successful people not only work hard, they also play hard. Childlike behavior generates joy, fun, and enthusiasm. Ask yourself: What can I do to stay in touch with my inner child?

Work Smart, Not Hard

Many caregivers never had the opportunity to learn essential time-management skills that result in working smart, not hard. You may find the following helpful:

• Create specific goals for personal and professional development. Break down your annual goals into monthly goals. Break down your weekly goals into daily goals. Ask yourself, "What do I want to accomplish this year, this month, this week, this day?" Planning each day can give you a road map to getting to your destination!

• Do one thing at a time. Caregivers are notorious for trying to do and be all things to all people and all projects all the time. Quality always suffer when you try to do too many things at once.

• End the day by planning tomorrow's projects whenever possible. That way, you'll not only waste less time getting started the following morning, you'll arrive at work feeling more in control of the day ahead.

• Protect yourself from constant interruptions. When you're working on a task, nothing will sabotage you more than interruptions. Block out the necessary time to complete tasks.

• Work when you work best. We all have certain natural peak hours of performance. Pay attention to your inner clock. Are you a morning person or a night person? Does a brief nap recharge you?

• Focus and reject. This is a reminder to stay focused on the task at hand. Learn to "switch off" those things that prevent you from accomplishing desired tasks. Sometimes this means delaying or returning calls and correspondence. If you always "stay available," you won't have time to accomplish what you may really want and need to accomplish.

- When all else fails, retreat to a hideout. When working on project development, you may need to find a "Skinner Box": a place where you can hole up with no interruptions. Tell only those who truly need to know where you are. You'll be amazed at what you get done.

- When you know your energy level is dropping, take a break. After a 10-minute walk or a short nap, you may be able to accomplish much more than you could have otherwise.

- Delegate tasks whenever possible. Watch out for "busy work" that might be done more efficiently by someone else.

- Throughout the day, ask yourself, "What's the best use of my time right now?" Focus on those tasks that need to be done first. This requires discipline, but will pay many dividends.

  Ask yourself, what am I doing to work smarter, not harder?

  _____
  _____
  _____
  _____
  _____
  _____

Build Support Systems

Our work requires a natural outward focus: on the needs of those we attempt to help. Such demands can leave us feeling emotionally and spiritually drained. An important aspect of self-care is to allow us to have sounding boards for how this work impacts our lives.

What do support systems provide for us? Ideally, supportive colleagues and friends provide some of the following:

Unconditional acceptance and support. In other words, friendships and the need to be nurtured and understood ourselves.

Help with complicated situations. Assistance in ideas that serve to help us in our efforts to help donor families.

Mentoring. Encouragement to continue to develop new tools to assist us in our work. Models that inspire us and remind us of the importance and value of our work.

Challenge. Encouragement to stretch ourselves beyond our current limits.

Referral. To have connection with additional resources for donor families in your care. Good caregivers will recognize occasions when it is appropriate to refer those we work with to other, rich sources of support and counsel.

> *Ask yourself, can I seek support systems when I need to? Who are the people in my life that make up my support system? List five people you could turn to right now for support and nurturing.*

_____

_____

_____

_____

_____

_____

_____

_____

_____

_____

Remember the Importance of "Spiritual Time"

We have found that nurturing our spirits is critical to our work as caregivers. "Spiritual time" helps us combat fatigue, frustration, and life's disappointments. To be present to those we work with and to learn from those we companion, we must appreciate the beauty of life and living.

Spiritual, quiet moments or "downtime" recharges spiritual energy. We encourage you to ask yourself: How do I renew my spirit?

Some people do this through prayer and meditation. Others might do this by hiking, biking, running, or other forms of physical alone time. Obviously, there is no one right way to renew your spirit. But one reality is that to be present to others in healing ways, we must each find a way to massage our spirits.

Consider the words of Carl Sandburg:

> A man must get away
>   now and then
>   to experience loneliness.
>
> Only those who learn how
>   to live in loneliness
>   can come to know themselves
>   and life.
>
> I go out there and walk
>   and look at the trees and sky.
> I listen to the sounds of loneliness.
> I sit on a rock or stump
>   and say to myself
>   "Who are you Sandburg?
>   Where have you been,
>   and where are you going?"

How do you keep your spirit alive? How do you listen to your heart? How do you appreciate the good, the beautiful, and the truthful in life?

_____

_____

_____

_____

_____

_____

Listen to Your Inner Voice

As a caregiver to the bereaved, you will at times become grief overloaded (too much death, grief, and loss in your day-to-day life). The natural demands of this kind of work can cause you to have tunnel vision about death and grief. For example, if your own child has a headache, you may immediately think brain tumor. If your partner complains of heartburn, you think heart attack.

Caregiving presents you with the gift of an enhanced awareness of the many tragedies that touch people's lives. Just as those you companion are changed by death, you are changed by their experiences as well. To embrace our deep appreciation for life and love we must stay grounded—and to do so means caring for ourselves as well as others.

Ask yourself, what is my own inner voice telling me about how to stay grounded?

_____

_____

_____

_____

_____

_____

A Self-Care Manifesto for Caregivers to the Bereaved

We who care for the bereaved have a wondrous opportunity: to help others embrace and grow through grief—and to lead fuller, more deeply-lived lives ourselves because of this important ministry.

But our work is draining—physically, emotionally, and spiritually. We must first care for ourselves if we want to care well for others. This manifesto is intended to empower you to practice good self-care.

1. *I deserve to lead a joyful, whole life. No matter how much I love and value my work, my life is multi-faceted. My family, my friends, my other interests, and my spirituality also deserve my time and attention. I deserve my time and attention.*

2. *My work does not define me. I am a unique, worthy person outside my work life. While relationships can help me feel good about myself, they are not what is inside me. Sometimes I need to stop "doing" and instead focus on simply "being."*

3. *I am not the only one who can help donor families. When I feel indispensable, I tend to ignore my own needs. There are many talented caregivers in my community who can also help the bereaved.*

4. *I must develop healthy eating, sleeping, and exercise patterns. I am aware of the importance of these things for those I help, but I may neglect them myself. A well-balanced diet, adequate sleep, and regular exercise allow me to be the best I can be.*

5. *If I've been over-involved in my caregiving for too long, I may have forgotten how to take care of myself. I may need to rediscover ways of caring for and nurturing myself. I may need to relearn how to explore my own feelings instead of focusing on everybody else's.*

6. *I must maintain boundaries in my helping relationships. As a caregiver, I cannot avoid getting emotionally involved with donor families. Nor would I want to. Active empathy allows me to be a good companion to them. However, I must remember I am responsible to others, not for others.*

7. *I am not perfect and I must not expect myself to be. I often wish my helping efforts were always successful. But even when I offer compassionate, "on-target" help, the recipient of that help isn't always prepared to use it. And when I do make mistakes, I should see them as an integral part of learning and growth, not as measurements of my self-worth.*

8. *I must practice effective time-management skills. I must set practical goals for how I spend my time. I must also remember Pareto's principle: twenty percent of what I do nets eighty percent of my results.*

9. *I must also practice setting limits and alleviating stresses I can do something about. I must work to achieve a clear sense of expectations and set realistic deadlines. I should enjoy what I do accomplish in helping others but shouldn't berate myself for what is beyond me.*

10. *I must listen to my inner voice. As a caregiver to donor families, I will at times become grief overloaded. When my inner voice begins to whisper its fatigue, I must listen carefully and allow myself some grief down-time.*

11. *I should express the personal me in both my work and play. I shouldn't be afraid to demonstrate my unique talents and abilities. I must also make time each day to remind myself of what is important to me. If I only had three months to live, what would I do?*

12. *I am a spiritual being. I must spend alone time focusing on self-understanding and self-love. To be present to those I work with and to learn from those I companion, I must appreciate the beauty of life and living. I must renew my spirit.*

Take time to summarize below the essential teaching principles you learned from reading the "After" section.

_____

_____

_____

_____

_____

_____

_____

_____

_____

A FINAL WORD

The opportunity to companion newly bereaved donor families is, without a doubt, a sacred experience. Our hope is that this resource will help you as a caregiver use your gifts to "companion," not "treat" those you are honored to walk with before, during, and after this difficult time.

It was Norman Cousins who said, "You will derive your supreme satisfaction...from your ability to identify yourself with others and to share fully in those needs and hopes." As you attempt to "share fully in the needs and hopes" of these families, you will be serving as a catalyst for a renewed sense of meaning and purpose in the lives of your fellow human beings. There is a wonderful line in Mitch Album's book *Tuesdays with Morrie*: "The most important thing in life is to learn how to give out love and let love come in." As you give out love to newly bereaved families, we know you will have love come in to your hearts and souls. Thanks for taking the time to read our effort to help you help co-create a meaningful donation experience families.

A Bill of Rights for Donor Families

This document is intended to represent the rights and legitimate expectations of families of loved ones who may die and may be considered potential organ and/or tissue donors. This document is also intended to serve as a guide for services that are or should be offered to such families. The term "family" identifies legal next-of-kin but is also intended to embrace other individuals who may have a significant relationship with a potential or actual organ and/or tissue donor, whether through biological, matrimonial, or affectional ties.

The term "donor family" identifies family members who may be or have already been approached to give consent for organ and/or tissue donation from the body of a loved one after death has occurred. This document does not address the situation of living persons who are contemplating or have consented to organ and/or tissue donation during their lifetime.

Bereaved donor families have the right:

1. *To a full and careful explanation about what has happened to their loved one, his or her current status, and his or her prognosis.*

2. *To be full partners with the healthcare team in the decision-making process about the care and support given to their loved one and to themselves.*

3. *To a full and careful explanation about the (impending) death of their loved one, with appropriate reference to the concept of cardiac and/or brain death and the basis upon which it has been or will be determined that that concept applies to their loved one.*

4. *To opportunities to be alone with their loved one during his or her care and after his or her death occurs. This should include offering the family an opportunity to see, touch, hold, or participate in the care of their loved one, as appropriate.*

5. *To be cared for in a manner that is sensitive to the family's needs and capacities by specially trained individuals.*

6. *To have an opportunity to make organ and/or tissue donation decisions on behalf of themselves and of their loved one who has died. This opportunity is to be included in the normal continuum of care by the healthcare provider after death has been determined and the family has had sufficient time to acknowledge that death has occurred.*

7. *To receive information in a manner that is suited to the family's needs and capacities about the need for organ and tissue donation, the conditions and processes of organ and/or tissue donation, and the implications of organ and/or tissue donation for later events,*

such as funeral arrangements, viewing of the body, and related practices.

8. *To be provided with time, privacy, freedom from coercion, confidentiality, and (if desired) the services of an appropriate support person (e.g., clergyperson) and other resources (e.g., a second medical opinion, advice from significant others, or the services of an interpreter for those who speak another language) which are essential to optimal care for the family and to enable family members to make an informed and free decision about donation.*

9. *To have their decisions about organ and/or tissue donation accepted and respected.*

10. *To have opportunities to spend time alone with their loved one before and/or after the process of removing donated organs and/or tissues, and to say their "good-byes" in a manner that is appropriate to the present and future needs of the family consistent with their cultural and religious identity (e.g., a lock of hair).*

11. *To be assured that their loved one will be treated with respect throughout the process of removing donated organs and/or tissues.*

12. *To receive timely information that is suited to the family's needs and capacities about which organs and/or tissues were or were not removed, and why.*

13. *To receive timely information regarding how any donated organs and/or tissues were used, and, if desired, to be given an opportunity to exchange anonymous communications with individual recipients and/or recipient family members. Upon request, donor families should also be given accurate updates on the condition of the recipients.*

14. *To be assured that the donor family will not be burdened with any expenses arising from organ and/or tissue donation, and to be given assistance in resolving any charges that might erroneously be addressed to the family.*

15. *To receive ongoing bereavement follow-up support for a reasonable period of time. Such support might take the form of: the name, address, and telephone number of a knowledgeable and sensitive person with whom they can discuss the entire experience; an opportunity to evaluate their experience through a quality assurance survey; free copies of literature about organ and/or tissue donation; free copies of literature about bereavement, grief, and mourning; opportunities for contact*

with another donor family; opportunities to take part in a donor or bereavement support group; and/or the services of a skilled and sensitive support person. All explanations mentioned in this document should be provided by a knowledgeable and sensitive person in a private, face-to-face conversation whenever possible in a manner suited to the family's needs. Also, these explanations may need to be repeated or supplemented in more than one interchange.

This Bill of Rights for Families has been officially endorsed by the following organizations:

> *North American Transplant Coordinators Organization*
> *Division of Transplantation Health Resources and Services Administration*
> *American Association of Critical-Care Nurses*
> *American Heart Association*
> *American Society of Transplant Physicians*

This document was prepared by:

> *Charles A. Corr, Ph.D., Lucy G. Nile, M.A. and the members of the National Donor Family Council of the National Kidney Foundation:*
> *Margaret B. Coolican, R.N., M.S. (Chairperson & donor family)*
> *William Bennett, M.D. (donor family)*
> *Vicki Crosier (donor family)*
> *Kenneth J. Doka, Ph.D. Jayne M. Miller (donor family)*
> *Kenneth Moritsugu, M.D., M.P.H. (donor family)*
> *Bea Olson (donor family)*
> *Therese A. Rando, Ph.D.*
> *Mark R. Reiner, P.A.*
> *Cynthia Rodriguez (donor family)*

NATIONAL DIRECTORY OF ORGAN AND TISSUE DONATION ORGANIZATIONS

American Association of Critical
Care Nurses (AACN)
101 Columbia
Aliso Viejo, CA 92656-4109
800.899.2226
www.aacn.org

American Association of Tissue Banks
(AATB)
1320 Old Chain Bridge Road
Suite 450
McLean, Virginia 22101
703-827-9582
Email: aatb@aatb.org
www.aatb.org

American Hospital Association (AHA)
155 N. Wacker Dr.
Chicago, Illinois 60606
312- 422-3000
800-242-2626
www.aha.org

American Medical Association (AMA)
515 N. State Street
Chicago, IL 60654
(800) 621-8335
www.ama-assn.org

American Red Cross
National Headquarters
2025 E Street, NW
Washington, DC 20006
(202) 303 – 5000
www.redcross.org

Association of Organ Procurement
Organizations (AOPO)
1364 Beverly Road, Suite 100,
McLean, VA 22101, USA
703 556-4242
Email: aopo@aopo.org
www.aopo.org

Children's Organ Transplant Association
(COTA)
2501 West COTA Drive
Bloomington, Indiana 47403
800.366.2682
Email: cota@cota.org

CoalitionOnDonation is now...
Donate Life America
700 N. Fourth Street
Richmond, Virginia 23219
804-782-4920
www.shareyourlife.org

Division of Transplantation at the
Dept of Health and Human Services
Parklawn Building
5600 Fishers Lane
Rockville, MD 20857
301.443.7577
www.organdonor.gov

Eye Bank Association of America
1015 Eighteenth Street NW, Suite 1010
Washington, DC 20036
202.775.4999
Email: info@restoresight.org
www.restoresight.org

The Living Bank
P. O. Box 6725
Houston, TX 77265-6725
1-800-528-2971
Email: info@livingbank.org
www.livingbank.org

The James Redford Institute
for Transplant Awareness
10573 West Pico Blvd., #214
Los Angeles, CA 90064-2348
310-559-6325
www.jrifilms.org

Musculoskeletal Transplant Foundation
(MTF)
125 May Street
Edison, NJ 08837
732-661-0202
800-433-6576
www.mtf.org

National Donor Family Council
30 East 33rd Street
New York, NY 10016
800-622-9010
www.kidney.org/transplantation/do-
norfamilies/index.cfm

National Kidney Foundation (NKF)
30 East 33rd Street
New York, NY 10016
1-800-622-9010
www.kidney.org

The Nicholas Green Foundation
5701 Alder Ridge Drive
La Cañada, CA 91011
E: green@nicholasgreen.org
818.952.2095

Minority Organ and Tissue Transplant
Education Progam (MOTTEP)
2041 Georgia Avenue, NW
Ambulatory Care Center, Suite 3100
Washington, D.C. 20060
(202) 865-4888
(800) 393-2839
www.mottep.org

The North American Transplant
Coordinators Organization (NATCO)
Executive Office
P.O. Box 15384
Lenexa, KS 66285-5384
913-895-4612
Email: natco-info@goAMP.com
http://www.natco1.org

South Eastern Organ Procurement
Foundation (SEOPF)
8154 Forest Hill Ave, Suite 3
Richmond, VA 23235
804- 323-9890
800- 543-6399
www.seopf.org

Transplant Recipients International
Organization, Inc. (TRIO)
2100 M Street, NW, #170-353
Washington, DC 20037-1233
800-TRIO-386
202- 293-0980
Email: info@trioweb.org
www.trioweb.org

Transweb
University of Michigan
Transplant Center
3868 Taubman Center
1500 E. Medical Center Drive, SPC
5391
Ann Arbor, Michigan 48109-5391
734-232-1113
Email: Transweb@umich.edu
TransWeb.org

United Network for Organ Sharing
(UNOS)
Corporate headquarters
Post Office Box 2484
Richmond, Virginia 23218
800.292.9548
888-894-6361
www.unos.org

NATIONAL BEREAVEMENT ORGANIZATIONS AND SUPPORT GROUPS

To receive a directory of support groups and services available for

Bereaved Children, contact:
  The Dougy Center
  P.O. Box 86852
  Portland, OR 97286
  (503) 775-5683
  www.dougy.org

For Widowed People:
  Widowed Persons Service
  Independent branches of this organization, formerly part of AARP, can be found by searching online for Widowed Persons Service and the name of your town or state.
  www.aarp.org

  THEOS
  (They Help Each Other Spiritually)
  322 Blvd. of the Allies #105
  Pittsburgh, PA 15222
  (412) 471-7799

For Parents Who Have Experienced the Death of a Child:
  The Compassionate Friends
  P.O. Box 3696
  Oak Brook, IL 60522-3696
  (603) 990-0010 or (877) 969-0010
  www.compassionatefriends.org

  Parents of Murdered Children
  100 East Eighth St., Suite 202
  Cincinnati, OH 45202
  (513) 721-5683 or (888) 818-POMC
  www.pomc.com

  Sudden Infant Death
  Syndrome Alliance
  1314 Bedford Ave., Suite 210
  Baltimore, MD 21208
  (800) 221-SIDS or (410) 653-8226
  www.firstcandle.org

American SIDS Institute
528 Raven Way
Naples, FL 34110
(239) 431-5425
www.sids.org

Candlelighters—American Childhood Cancer Organization
P.O. Box 498
Kensington, MD 20895
(800) 366-2223
www.candlelighters.org

For Miscarriage, Stillbirth, Ectopic Pregnancy and Early Infant Death:
  International Council on Infertility Information Dissemination (INCIID)
  P.O. Box 6836
  Arlington, VA 22206
  (703) 379-9178
  www.inciid.org

  Share National Office
  401 Jackson Street
  St. Charles, MO 63301-2893
  (636) 947-6164 or (800) 821-6819
  www.nationalshare.org

For Homicide:
  Mothers Against Drunk Driving (MADD)
  511 E. John Carpenter Freeway
  Suite 700
  Irving, TX 75062
  (800) GET-MADD
  www.MADD.org

  National Organization For Victim Assistance (NOVA)
  510 King Street, Suite 424
  Alexandria, VA 22314
  (703) 535-NOVA or (800) TRY-NOVA
  www.trynova.org

Safe Horizon
2 Lafayette St.
New York, NY 10007
24-hour Hotline: (800) 621-HOPE
www.safehorizon.org

For Suicide:
American Association
of Suicidology
5221 Wisconsin Avenue, NW
Washington, DC 20015
(202) 237-2280
National Suicide Prevention Lifeline:
(800) 273-TALK
www.suicidology.org

The Samaritans
141 Tremont St., 7th Floor
Boston, MA 02111
(617) 247-0220
(800) 252-8336
www.samaritansofboston.org

For Hospice Care:
National Hospice and Palliative
Care Organization
1731 King Street, Suite 100
Alexandria, VA 22314
(703) 837-1500
www.caringinfo.org

For AIDS:
AIDS Action
1730 M Street NW
Suite 611
Washington, DC 20036
(202) 530-8030
www.aidsaction.org

For Support Groups:
National Mental Health Consumers'
Self-Help Clearinghouse
1211 Chestnut Street, Suite 1207
Philadelphia, PA 19107
(215) 751-1810
(800) 553-4539
www.mhselfhelp.org

For Bereavement Care Training
Opportunities:
The Center for Loss and
Life Transition
3735 Broken Bow Road
Fort Collins, CO 80526
(970) 226-6050
www.centerforloss.com

AUTHOR WORKSHOPS
AND TRAININGS

Dr. Raelynn Maloney and Dr. Alan Wolfelt are available to present workshops and trainings to hospital staff, organ or tissue procurement staff, call center staff, and area caregivers on caring for donor families. Public presentations for the bereaved on coping with grief and loss are also available. Formats offered include all-day workshops, breakfast or dinner presentations, keynote addresses, in-house staff trainings and consultations following difficult cases.

One of today's most respected and popular educators, Dr. Alan Wolfelt is also a grief companion and author. He serves as director of the Center for Loss and Life Transition in Fort Collins, Colorado and is on the faculty at the University of Colorado Medical School's Department of Family Medicine. Dr. Wolfelt has become a "responsible rebel" who advocates for grief care that is compassionate, mourner-led and soul- and spirit-based.

Dr. Raelynn Maloney has worked with bereaved families and caregivers who support donor families since 1994. She is currently a licensed psychologist working in private practice in Littleton, Colorado. As an author, educator and counselor, Raelynn provides consultation to OPOs, Tissuebanks, hospitals, and funeral directors on a variety of topics related to grief, loss, and organ/tissue donation.

For more information on sponsoring a workshop in your area, please call the Center for Loss at 970.226.6050.

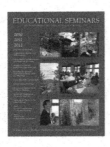

ATTENTION BEREAVEMENT CAREGIVERS!

Have you heard about the great courses taught by Dr. Wolfelt at the Center for Loss in Fort Collins, Colorado? He offers 4-day seminars on the following topics:

- Comprehensive Bereavement Skills Training
- Understanding and Responding to Complicated Mourning
- Helping Children and Adolescents Cope with Grief
- Exploring the Spiritual Dimensions of Death, Grief and Mourning
- Counseling Skills Fundamentals
- Living with Meaning and Purpose in Your Life
- Support Group Facilitator Training
- Suicide Grief: Companioning the Mourner
- Companioning the Dying (with Greg Yoder)
- Funeral Service Enrichment Experience
- Exploring the Shadow of the Ghosts of Grief
- Pet Loss Companioning Certification Program

An accredited certification in Death & Grief Studies is also available.

For more information, please visit www.centerforloss.com or call us at 970.226.6050 to request a complete course catalog.

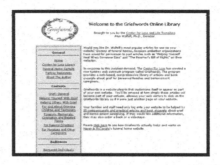

GRIEFWORDS

Check it out at
griefwords.com & horanandmcconaty.com

The Center for Loss has created a great turnkey web outreach program called Griefwords. The program provides a web-based, comprehensive library of articles and book excerpts (56 in all!) about grief for bereaved families and bereavement caregivers.

How does it work?
Griefwords is a website plug-in, not a website. If your website does not already contain a section on bereavement or aftercare, Griefwords will provide you with a complete library of information. If your website contains a section on bereavement or aftercare, Griefwords can become an integral part of the section you have already created.

How do I subscribe?
To subscribe to Griefwords, please call us or fax us your order by listing Griefwords on the enclosed order form. We'll contact you within 3 business days to get the additional information we need to install the Griefwords plug-in.

Griefwords Web Outreach Program
$450 first year subscription
$150/year renewal thereafter

ALSO BY DR. ALAN WOLFELT
AND DR. RAELYNN MALONEY

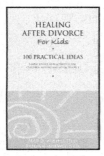

Healing After Divorce:
100 Practical Ideas for Kids

by Alan D. Wolfelt, Ph.D. and
Raelynn Maloney, Ph.D.

While divorce is common, it's also very difficult for
children, eliciting many challenging feelings. This book for
kids 7-12 gives them 100 simple ideas for expressing their
emotions during this life-changing time so that they can go
on to lead happy lives and develop healthy relationships of
their own.

ISBN 978-1-61722-138-5 • softcover • 128 pages • $11.95

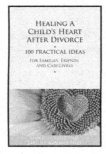

Healing A Child's Heart
After Divorce
100 Practical Ideas for Families,
Friends and Caregivers

by Alan D. Wolfelt, Ph.D. and
Raelynn Maloney, Ph.D.

How do you help children whose parents are separated or
divorced? While divorce represents a significant loss for
children—a loss that creates all the many natural feelings of
grief, the children can continue to thrive if they are helped in these 100 practical
ways by the caring adults in their lives.

ISBN 978-1-61722-142-2 • softcover • 128 pages • $11.95

ALSO BY DR. ALAN WOLFELT

THE SUICIDE GRIEF TRILOGY

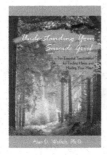

Understanding Your Suicide Grief

Using the metaphor of the wilderness, Dr. Wolfelt introduces ten Touchstones that will assist the survivor in what is often a complicated grief journey. Learning to identify and rely on the Touchstones helps those touched by suicide find their way to hope and healing.

ISBN 978-1-879651-58-6 • 194 pages • softcover • $14.95

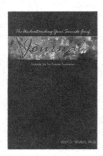

The Understanding Your Suicide Grief Journal

This companion journal to *Understanding Your Suicide Grief* helps you explore the ten essential Touchstones for finding hope and healing your grieving heart after the suicide death of someone loved. Throughout, you'll be reminded of the content you have read in the companion book and asked corresponding questions about your profound, unique grief.

ISBN 978-1-879651-59-3 • 136 pages • softcover • $14.95

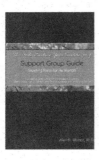

The Understanding Your Suicide Grief Support Group Guide
Meeting Plans for Facilitators

This book is for those who want to facilitate an effective suicide grief support group. It includes 12 meeting plans that interface with *Understanding Your Suicide Grief* and its companion journal.

ISBN 978-1-879651-60-9 • 44 pages • softcover • $12.95

ALSO BY DR. ALAN WOLFELT

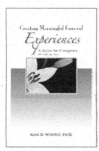

Creating Meaningful Funeral Experiences

A Guide for Caregivers

This revised, updated version of Dr. Wolfelt's groundbreaking *Creating Meaningful Funeral Ceremonies* includes current statistics as well as an introduction to the concept of funerals not just as ceremonies, but as experiences. The book explores the ways in which personalized funerals transform mourners. It also reviews qualities in caregivers that make them effective celebrants and funeral planners and provides practical. ideas for creating authentic, personalized and meaningful funeral experiences.

ISBN 978-1-879651-38-8 • 80 pages • softcover • $12.95

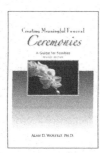

Creating Meaningful Funeral Ceremonies

A Guide for Families

This compassionate, friendly workbook affirms the importance of the personalized funeral ritual and helps families create a ceremony that will be both healing and meaningful for years to come. Designed to complement the role of the clergy, celebrant and funeral director in the funeral planning process, *A Guide for Families* walks readers through the many decisions they will make at the time of a death.

ISBN 978-1-879651-20-3 • 80 pages • softcover • $12.95

Special Set Price: Order both *Creating Meaningful Ceremonies* books for more than 20% off! Set - $20.00

ALSO BY DR. ALAN WOLFELT

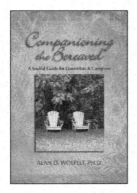

Companioning the Bereaved
A Soulful Guide for Caregivers
by Alan D. Wolfelt, Ph.D.

This book by one of North America's most respected grief educators presents a model for grief counseling based on his "companioning" principles.

For many mental healthcare providers, grief in contemporary society has been medicalized—perceived as if it were an illness that with proper assessment, diagnosis and treatment could be cured.

Dr. Wolfelt explains that our modern understanding of grief all too often conveys that at bereavement's "end" the mourner has completed a series of tasks, extinguished pain, and established new relationships. Our psychological models emphasize "recovery" or "resolution" in grief, suggesting a return to "normalcy."

By contrast, this book advocates a model of "companioning" the bereaved, acknowledging that grief forever changes or transforms the mourner's world view. Companioning is not about assessing, analyzing, fixing or resolving another's grief. Instead, it is about being totally present to the mourner, even being a temporary guardian of his soul. The companioning model is grounded in a "teach me" perspective.

"This outstanding book should be required reading for each and every grief provider. Dr. Wolfelt's philosophy and practice of caregiving helps us understand we don't need to be joined at the head with the mourner, we need to be joined at the heart."
— Grief Counselor

ISBN 978-1-879651-41-8 • hardcover • 176 pages • $29.95

ALSO BY DR. ALAN WOLFELT

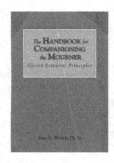

The Handbook for Companioning the Mourner
Eleven Essential Principles

This inspiring handbook explores Dr. Wolfelt's "companioning" model of grief care and contrasts it with the traditional "treatment" model. Concise and engaging, this is a primer designed to spread the companioning philosophy among everyone who walks alongside mourners—counselors, hospice caregivers, funeral home staff, friends and family members.

Join the companioning movement, which is transforming our mourning-avoidant North American culture into one that embraces the normal, necessary and transformative journey through grief.

Caregivers around the world are talking about the companioning model of grief care:

"Dr. Wolfelt's companioning philosophy resonates with my spirit and makes my heart sing."

"Finally, a model of caregiving that is inherently compassionate and heart-based, not head-based."

"I have put this philosophy of care into action and been amazed at the results."

"We need to advocate for this model of care throughout the world. I'm going to get these loving tenets into the hands of as many people as I possibly can."

"I attended the training on this model of caregiving at Dr. Wolfelt's Center for Loss and returned home humbled and touched by my experience. Thank you so much for your efforts to humanize the care of people wounded by loss and grief."

ISBN 978-1-879651-61-6 • 128 pages • hardcover • $15.95

ALSO BY DR. ALAN WOLFELT

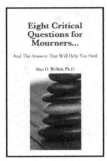

Eight Critical Questions for Mourners...
And the Answers That Will Help You Heal

When loss enters your life, you are faced with many choices. The questions you ask and the choices you make will determine whether you become among the "living dead" or go on to live until you die. If you are going to integrate grief into your life, it helps to recognize what questions to ask yourself on the journey.

1. Will I grieve or mourn this loss?

2. Will I befriend my feelings of loss, or will I inhibit them?

3. Will I be a passive witness or an active participant in my grief?

4. Will I embrace the uniqueness of my grief?

5. Will I work on the six needs of mourning, or will I fall victim to the cliché "time heals all wounds?"

6. Will I believe I must achieve resolution, or will I work toward reconciliation?

7. Will I embrace my transformation?

8. Will this loss add to my "divine spark" or will it take away my life force?

This book provides the answers that will help you clarify your experiences and encourage you to make choices that honor the transformational nature of grief and loss.

ISBN 978-1-879651-62-3 • 176 pages • softcover • $18.95

ALSO BY DR. ALAN WOLFELT

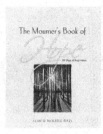

The Mourner's Book of Hope

To integrate loss and to move forward with a life of meaning and love, you must have hope. Hope is a belief in a good that is yet to be. This beautiful little hardcover gift book offers Dr. Wolfelt's thoughts on hope in grief interspersed with quotes from the world's greatest hope-filled thinkers.

When we become aware that we do not have to escape our pains,
but that we can mobilize them into a common search for life,
those very pains are transformed from expressions
of despair into signs of hope.
- Henri Nouwen

Hope begins in the dark,
the stubborn hope that if you just show up
and try to do the right thing,
the dawn will come.
You wait and watch and work:
you don't give up.
- Anne Lamott

Hope and hopelessness are both choices.
Why not choose hope?
- Greg Anderson

ISBN 978-1-879651-65-4 • 200 pages
hardcover • $15.95

ALSO BY DR. ALAN WOLFELT

FOR BEREAVEMENT
SUPPORT GROUPS

Understanding Your Grief and its companion journal
and guide for support group leaders are among
Dr. Wolfelt's most well-known and -used books.
Together the three provide a compassionate philosophy and
comprehensive framework for both support group members and leaders.

For bereavement support group leaders and participants, this package contains
two copies of *The Understanding Your Grief Support Group Guide* and ten copies
each of *Understanding Your Grief* and *The Understanding Your Grief Journal*.
Subsequent orders of 10 or more copies of *Understanding Your Grief* and the
journal receive a 15% discount.

Support Group Start-up Package • $270

"*As a bereavement support group leader, I've found that the*
Understanding Your Grief *trilogy provides me with a very user-friendly framework and helps me create a safe place for mourners to
learn about and explore their grief.*"
— Charles (Duke) Quarles, US Navy Chaplain